BREASTFEEDING POSITIVELY

ESSENTIAL INFORMATION FOR MOTHERS LIVING WITH HIV

BREASTFEEDING POSITIVELY

ESSENTIAL INFORMATION FOR MOTHERS LIVING WITH HIV

PAMELA MORRISON

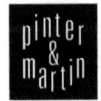

Breastfeeding Positively: Essential Information for Mothers Living with HIV

First published by Pinter & Martin Ltd 2024

© 2024 Pamela Morrison

The author has asserted her moral rights to be identified as the author of this work in accordance with the Copyright, Designs and Patents Act of 1988.

All rights reserved

ISBN 978-1-78066-805-5

Also available as ebook

Editor Susan Last

Index by Helen Bilton

British Library Cataloguing-in-Publication Data
A catalogue record for this book is available from the British Library.

This book is sold subject to the condition that it shall not, by way of trade and otherwise, be lent, resold, hired out, or otherwise circulated without the publisher's prior consent in any form or binding or cover other than that in which it is published and without a similar condition being imposed on the subsequent purchaser.

Pinter & Martin
Unit 803 Omega Works
4 Roach Road
London E3 2PH

pinterandmartin.com

CONTENTS

Disclaimer	6

Section I: Choosing to breastfeed with HIV

1. Introduction	8
2. The research on HIV and breastfeeding	16
3. Advance planning and enlisting help	32
4. The transformational effect of antiretroviral therapy	48
5. Why exclusive breastfeeding matters	52

Section I: How breastfeeding works

6. Beginning breastfeeding, positioning and attachment, latching techniques	62
7. Lactation management for mothers	83
8. Mixed breastfeeding after six months	102
9. Weaning from the breast	109
10. Expressing, pumping, storing breastmilk, and feeding breastmilk	118
11. Pasteurising/flash-heating	130

Section III: Troubleshooting

12. Breast problems	138
13. Nipple problems	149
14. Breastfeeding problems: supplementing, suspending and transitioning back	165
15. Suppression of lactation	188
16. Conclusion	194
Acknowledgements	196
References	198
Index	217

Disclaimer

Information in this book about breastfeeding with HIV (how to plan for, initiate and maintain breastfeeding as safely and successfully as possible) should not be construed as medical advice. It is not intended to replace the personal guidance that a mother should obtain from her own HIV clinician, obstetrician, paediatrician, general practitioner/medical doctor, midwives and other healthcare providers. Ultimately, decisions relating to your treatment and your baby's health should always be taken in consultation with the doctor or other trained healthcare worker who knows you, your baby and your special medical care needs.

You can discuss the research on breastfeeding with HIV within these pages with your doctors (especially the information in Chapter 2), so that clinicians can assess whether the strategies offered to facilitate breastfeeding are safe. At the same time, as a mother living with HIV you can ask that medical advice can be tailored to your specific circumstances so that you can achieve your own goals, whether that is breastfeeding for a short time, or a long time, and so that when you and your baby are ready, you can stop breastfeeding easily and safely.

Some of the techniques and protocols for nipple and breast care, and how to resolve common difficulties laid out in chapters 12, 13 and 14, are based on my own observation and practice as a lactation consultant. They have been developed and honed over several years, by observing what worked for individual mothers. Once again, these suggestions are not to be construed as medical advice.

SECTION I

CHOOSING TO BREASTFEED WITH HIV

1. INTRODUCTION

Mothers living with HIV want to breastfeed

Mothers living with HIV in high-income countries are showing more interest than ever before in breastfeeding their babies. Today we have research showing that mothers' own milk poses a much lower risk of HIV transmission than they have been previously led to believe. When they hear about it, many are interested in finding out what it might mean for them and their babies (See Chapter 2.)

A very large percentage of women living with HIV have arrived in First World countries from areas of high HIV prevalence, especially in Africa, where global recommendations supporting breastfeeding are followed due to better health outcomes compared to formula-feeding. Back home, where these mothers grew up (as I did myself) breastfeeding was an integral part of Africa's traditions and culture since time immemorial. Becoming a mother elevates a woman's status in society and breastfeeding her babies is both a duty and a privilege. Breastfeeding is culturally normal and keeps babies healthy.

In spite of strong efforts around the turn of the millennium by the international health agencies to prevent HIV transmission through breastfeeding by encouraging mothers with HIV to formula-feed, Africa is probably the last continent in the world to embrace breastmilk substitutes. Most babies still enjoy the health advantages of being breastfed well into their second year of life. This is in stark contrast to feeding norms in the West, where breasts have become sexualised, and formula-feeding seems normal so that mothers living with HIV feel pressured *not* to breastfeed, causing stigma and much distress.

Past research

Research conducted in the first decade of the new millennium showed clearly that in the context of HIV, more babies who were breastfed survived to grow up than those who were formula-fed. In 2009, global guidance that had previously promoted formula to avoid postpartum HIV-transmission[1] was reversed.[2] African mothers today, whether they have HIV or not, are urged to exclusively breastfeed for the first six months and continue partial breastfeeding for up to two years or beyond.[3] Consequently, their expectation of breastfeeding their babies has not dimmed just because they may now be living in the First World, with a diagnosis of HIV. They retain their friends, their networks and their cultural traditions when they emigrate. Breastfeeding is important to African mothers whether they live in Kenya, Khayelitsha or Kensington.

However, contradictory cultural values create a dilemma in infant feeding advice. And it is this which underpins the writing of this book especially for mothers with HIV who wish to breastfeed. Formula-feeding is seen as so normal in many First World countries that we may be losing the ability to support women with breastfeeding.[4]

One of my clever and articulate clients shared with me that although her HIV clinicians wanted to support her infant feeding choice, none of them had actually worked with a breastfeeding mother before. This meant that they had limited practical knowledge to offer. This mother's confidence was frequently undermined by her paediatrician's concerns about the risk of HIV transmission through breastfeeding, exacerbated by uncertainty about what might be normal. The paediatrician criticised the mother's wish to respond to her baby's frequent, yet entirely normal, 24/7 feeding cues. Wouldn't short feeding intervals 'spoil' the baby? Shouldn't the baby be sleeping through the night by now? Could mother's milk alone fulfil the baby's nutritional needs for a full six months? Wouldn't the baby need formula supplements? Shouldn't she start complementary feeding at four months instead of six? Since the baby was healthy, happy and gaining weight well, the mother managed to resist these suggestions. But worryingly, while the paediatrician was fretting about liability due to any breastfeeding, mixed breast and formula-feeding for a baby under six months is a risk factor for mother-to-child transmission of HIV, requiring weaning, so this unhelpful advice seemed contrived to sabotage the mother's wish to continue breastfeeding, rather than protect the baby's health.

When British breastfeeding rates are among the lowest in the world, and the healthcare providers of only one in 100 babies will have had experience with babies who are fed according to global infant feeding recommendations, either in or out of the context of HIV, it's entirely understandable that breastfeeding is viewed with a certain measure of suspicion. Nevertheless, when mothers living with HIV have their hearts set on breastfeeding, there is an obligation on us to help them succeed.

This book is written, then, for mothers living with HIV who want to breastfeed. The aim is to provide you with topics to discuss with your doctors so that you can make an informed decision. It provides:

- background information about the normal course of lactation
- 'how-to' information to initiate and maintain breastfeeding
- how to prevent, work through or around the difficulties that arise
- how to maintain breastmilk production or breastmilk-feeding if supplements should be recommended, including strategies so that you don't have to stop breastfeeding completely in order to avoid 'mixed feeding'.

The book is written especially through an HIV lens – to provide strategies to make breastfeeding with HIV possible and to cut through some of the 'myth-information' which mothers receive from other sources. It contains tips and techniques to avoid some of the common pitfalls that beset so many breastfeeding mothers living in industrialised countries, as well as ways to overcome them while working with your healthcare providers to keep your baby healthy.

If, in consultation with your HIV specialists, obstetrician and paediatrician, you decide to go ahead, breastfeeding with HIV requires a few extra considerations. This book suggests ways to take a little extra care. Anticipatory care tailored to these special challenges can help to avoid most difficulties before they arise, and to work through or around them if they happen. If you are a mother living with HIV who wants to breastfeed, then this book is for you.

About me

What experience do I bring to the subject of breastfeeding with HIV? I'm not medically trained, but as a volunteer breastfeeding counsellor for La Leche League since 1987 and then as a candidate for the International Board of Lactation Consultant Examiners (IBLCE) exam in 1990 I was required to study and had clocked 2,500 supervised hours working with breastfeeding mothers and babies. Since then I have racked up over 35 years' experience helping approximately 3,500 mother-baby pairs to breastfeed in both routine and special circumstances. In 2003, Zimbabwe had the highest rate of HIV infection in the world, with 30% of pregnant women testing positive, so the question of breastfeeding with HIV was increasingly raised.

My clients came from all nationalities, races, and ethnicities and their babies ranged in age from one hour to 6½ years of age. Having hospital privileges meant that I was able to work with mothers of newborns to assist them with initiating breastfeeding shortly after birth, and then to offer home or office visits once mother and baby went home from the hospital. Since exclusive breastfeeding from birth and for the first six months was the national recommendation, infant formula was simply not available in the maternity units for full-term healthy babies. All healthcare providers spoke with one voice, and it was essential that the babies were able to establish breastfeeding because their paediatricians would not discharge them home until they were either breastfeeding effectively, or mothers were able to express and cup-feed enough breastmilk for them to thrive.

I was also able to see pre-term babies in the Neonatal Intensive Care Unit, the youngest and smallest being surviving twins of a triplet pregnancy born at 26 weeks weighing 600g and 700g who were able to go home 100 days later exclusively breastmilk-fed. Healthy preemie babies were usually discharged home exclusively breastfeeding at 34 weeks or when they reached 1,800g, whichever was the later, so maternal motivation to provide their own milk and then to begin breastfeeding was high.

I received referrals, and was mentored by the very dedicated obstetricians and paediatricians who worked to protect, promote and support breastfeeding in Zimbabwe's very baby-friendly culture. Initiation of breastfeeding was almost 100%. Ninety-three percent of babies were still breastfeeding into their second year. Working in a country where breastfeeding was so well promoted and supported was a unique experience. I was a practitioner, and there was little need for breastfeeding advocacy. We had a National Breastfeeding Co-ordinator at the Ministry of Health who ensured that breastfeeding was kept on everyone's agenda. Legislation was in place to provide maternity leave and nursing breaks for working mothers, and there were large countrywide celebrations every year to mark World Breastfeeding Week. I served on the National Breastfeeding Committee, on the Baby-Friendly Task Force, and on committees to draft Code legislation (which prevented the inappropriate marketing of breastmilk substitutes) and to develop HIV and breastfeeding policy.

My first HIV+ client was referred to me by La Leche League in December 1995. The mother had just tested positive on an HIV test, and her doctor had advised her to wean her eight-month-old baby immediately to prevent him contracting the virus. The mother was terribly distressed, both because of the diagnosis and because the baby was refusing a bottle. During extensive attempts to access information for this young mother, I realised that very little was known about breastfeeding with HIV. Breastfeeding is important to all mothers and in a developing country breastfeeding may be life-saving. Since then, my special interest has focused on how the risk of transmission is assessed and how that risk can be minimised.

In 2003 our family emigrated to Australia and within two years we moved again to England. Between 2005 and 2018 I was employed by the World Alliance for Breastfeeding Action (WABA) as a consultant on HIV and breastfeeding. I was the main author of a set of documents called the HIV Kit, which was published in 2012 and updated in 2018.[5]

I officially registered as Retired with the IBLCE Examining Board at the end of 2020, but I continue to work as a volunteer to support mothers living with HIV who want to breastfeed and I advocate where I can for clarity in guidance. In February 2022, Pinter & Martin published my book *HIV and Breastfeeding: The Untold Story*, which tells the tale of how, due to HIV, breastfeeding almost became an endangered practice.[6]

Definitions

When reading research about HIV and breastfeeding, definitions can be crucial. Sloppy descriptions can cause confusion, and may even be dangerous. We must know what we are talking about, because who feeds what to an HIV-exposed baby can make the difference between life and death.

Women living with HIV who become mothers are often described as *mothers living with HIV*, and they in turn are often described in the literature as *HIV-positive mothers, HIV+ mothers, or HIV-infected mothers*. This terminology may be used in this book for brevity, and there is no disrespect intended.

In the African countries I grew up in and lived in for most of my life, becoming a mother elevated a woman's status in society. Motherhood bestowed on women a special place in the community, even as it handed her many obligations. In the interests of clarity, I refer to the mother as 'she' and the baby as 'he' throughout most of this book.

In the absence of preventative measures, babies can contract HIV from their mothers during pregnancy, during birth or during breastfeeding. Without wishing to blame mothers, this phenomenon is often described as *mother-to-child transmission (MTCT)*, or *vertical transmission (VT)*. When transmission occurs during pregnancy it is described as *antenatal transmission, prenatal transmission* or *pregnancy-associated transmission*. When transmission occurs through breastfeeding, it is sometimes called *postpartum transmission (PP transmission)*. The term *parent-to-child transmission* is less clear, since HIV cannot be passed directly to babies by their fathers, so it will not be used in this text.

The way *breastfeeding* is described is especially important. The protective effect of breastfeeding on the severity and duration of any disease is directly influenced by the exclusivity of breastfeeding, and HIV is no exception. Older research which apparently demonstrates that 'breastfeeding' transmits HIV often fails to describe whether the researchers mean:

- *any breastfeeding* (even once a day, or once only)
- *partial breastfeeding* (for a short time, or only occasionally)
- *predominant breastfeeding* (almost all breastfeeding but with the occasional addition of other milks)
- *mixed breastfeeding* (breastmilk and formula-feeding, or other complementary foods)
- *exclusive breastfeeding* (mother's milk only, with absolutely nothing else other than medically prescribed medications).
- *feeding* (colloquial abbreviation for 'breastfeeding' used in English-speaking countries like the UK, Australia and New Zealand)
- *infant feeding* (UN agencies' terminology used to describe breastfeeding, but may also mean any food or liquid fed to a baby).

Crucially, *exclusive breastfeeding for the first six months of life* poses the least risk of breastfeeding-associated transmission of the HIV virus.

Mixed breastfeeding after six months (with the normal and gradual addition of other complementary foods and liquids during the normal slow weaning process) does not carry the same risk of transmission as it does when babies are prematurely exposed to foreign substances (this will be further discussed in Chapter 8 on mixed feeding.)

For the purposes of scrutinising research on HIV and infant

feeding, it is necessary to take great care to ascertain exactly what the baby is being fed. It can be seen from these descriptions that 'infant feeding' or even just 'feeding' are terms that can mean many things to many people, and can cover a multitude of indiscretions:

- Is the mother exclusively breastfeeding the baby?
- Is the baby receiving other feeds of other milks or other liquids?
- Is a grandmother giving the baby prelacteal feeds – little sips of water or other traditional foods?
- Is an HIV+ transgender father chest-feeding?
  > has he had a mastectomy and
  > does this mean feeding formula through a nursing supplementer?
- Is a mother or caregiver topping the baby up with formula supplements or extra sips of water, and if so
  > when did they start,
  > for how long did they last, and
  > when did all breastfeeding end?
- Has the mother breastfed directly at the breast?
- Has the mother fed her expressed her milk to the baby so that he has in fact been breastmilk-fed, or partly breastmilk and partly formula-fed?
- Has the baby under six months been prematurely fed with other solid foods?

All of these scenarios can impact the integrity of the baby's gut, which in turn will affect the risk of transmission of the virus. How transparent is the conclusion reached? What does this mean for the outcome of a piece of research reported, or reviewed, or included in a meta-analysis of many papers added together? If only it was clear that one feeding method carried risks and another didn't – but it's not that simple. As we shall see in Chapter 5 on exclusive breastfeeding, when you're deciding how to feed your baby, definitions can make all the difference.

15

2. THE RESEARCH ON HIV AND BREASTFEEDING

Why breastfeeding matters

Mothers living with HIV who are considering breastfeeding their babies generally, and wisely, find out all they can before the birth of their babies, or sometimes even before they become pregnant, so that they have plenty of time to weigh the issues and decide what they want to do.

Outside the context of HIV, mothers are mindful that breastfeeding receives good publicity. The health advantages of breastfeeding are well promoted and undisputed.[1]

Risks and benefits

WHO recommends that mothers living with HIV should also breastfeed while receiving antiretroviral therapy, exclusively for the first six months, and with the addition of appropriate weaning foods to 24 months.[2] But for these mothers living in the UK and other First World countries, the guidance is sometimes different. While they receive health messages extolling the importance of breastfeeding generally, they also receive targeted warnings about how HIV can sometimes be transmitted through breastmilk. This poses a dilemma; even though the risk of transmission may be low, if it occurs in a single case, the consequences of HIV transmission are life-long. So while the advantages are a given, what mothers want to know – and need to think about carefully – is how much of a risk breastfeeding poses in terms of HIV transmission. Which feeding method – breastfeeding or formula-feeding – is going to be the healthiest and safest for their babies, in their individual circumstances? It's a big decision and the answer is not always straightforward.

WHO overview and recommendations on breastfeeding

Over the past decades, evidence for the health advantages of breastfeeding and recommendations for practice have continued to increase. WHO can now say with full confidence that breastfeeding reduces child mortality and has health benefits that extend into adulthood. On a population basis, exclusive breastfeeding for the first six months of life is the recommended way of feeding infants, followed by continued breastfeeding with appropriate complementary foods for up to two years or beyond.

To enable mothers to establish and sustain exclusive breastfeeding for six months, WHO and UNICEF recommend:

- *Initiation of breastfeeding within the first hour of life;*
- *Exclusive breastfeeding - that is, the infant only receives breastmilk without any additional food or drink, not even water;*
- *Breastfeeding on demand - that is, as often as the child wants, day and night;*
- *No use of bottles, teats or pacifiers.*

Breastmilk is the natural first food for babies, it provides all the energy and nutrients that the infant needs for the first months of life, and it continues to provide up to half or more of a child's nutritional needs during the second half of the first year, and up to one-third during the second year of life.

Breastmilk promotes sensory and cognitive development, and protects the infant against infectious and chronic diseases. Exclusive breastfeeding reduces infant mortality due to common childhood illnesses such as diarrhoea or pneumonia, and helps for a quicker recovery during illness.

Breastfeeding contributes to the health and well-being of mothers, it helps to space children, reduces the risk of ovarian cancer and breast cancer, increases family and national resources, is a secure way of feeding and is safe for the environment.

Cultural norms

Each individual mother brings to her pregnancy her unique personal background and current circumstances. Mothers have heard about the latest research confirming that breastfeeding with HIV is safer than it used to be[3] and that bonding with the baby is easier than if they bottle-feed formula. Additionally, the largest percentage of mothers living with HIV in the UK and other First World countries have usually emigrated from areas where HIV prevalence is high, especially eastern, central and southern Africa. Furthermore, they bring their traditions and cultural norms with them. Back home, breastfeeding is highly valued. Mothers worry that formula-feeding will reveal their HIV status to others in their community, exposing them to severe stigma, because why else would you *not* want to breastfeed? If they must bottle-feed they sometimes do it in secret because not breastfeeding is so shameful. Breastfeeding is important for all sorts of reasons, and women can be eloquent in describing feelings of sadness, grief and shame when they've been prevented from breastfeeding previous babies. Fortunately things are changing, and today most current national recommendations specify that while formula-feeding is usually recommended, mothers who want to breastfeed should also be supported to do so.

The research background

Although there is no such thing as zero risk in any endeavour, the research available today shows that under certain conditions, which are not difficult to achieve, the risk of infecting a baby with HIV through breastfeeding can be reduced to virtually nil. Later chapters in this book outline practical suggestions so that mothers can fulfil their dream of breastfeeding while at the same time keeping their babies as safe as possible.

But in the past, things were much more difficult. Almost as soon as the first report from Australia was released in 1985 showing that HIV could be passed to a baby through breastfeeding,[4] the industrialised countries moved quickly to effectively ban breastfeeding by mothers who had acquired the virus. It took almost a decade longer for effective antiretroviral therapy (ART) to be available. Because bottle-feeding was seen as normal and safe, exposing babies to the risk of acquiring HIV through mother's milk was seen as unnecessary.

Towards the end of the 1990s, in an effort to reduce the number of babies becoming infected through breastfeeding, the international health agencies, UNAIDS, WHO and UNICEF, began to offer counselling and free infant formula to HIV+ mothers in developing countries. Women received testing in early pregnancy; those testing positive were offered short-course ART and counselling about 'replacement feeding', i.e. how to feed their babies formula. The rationale behind this initiative, which continues to influence doctors and clinicians in First World countries today, said:

> *When children born to women living with HIV can be ensured uninterrupted access to nutritionally adequate breast-milk substitutes that are safely prepared and fed to them, they are at less risk of illness and death if they are not breast-fed.*[5]

However, in resource-poor settings without safe, piped water or easy access to medical care, hospitals and antibiotics, withholding breastfeeding placed babies at risk for malnutrition and mortality due to common childhood infections, especially pneumonia and diarrhoea. Researchers started to look at 'HIV-free survival' instead, and in 2009 WHO reversed the advice not to breastfeed.[6]

The advent of antiretroviral therapy (ART)

The development of effective antiretroviral therapy[7] has turned HIV from a dreaded lethal disease which inevitably led to death due to AIDS, to a chronic, inconvenient but manageable condition, like diabetes. From 1994 onwards, researchers began offering short courses of ART to nursing mothers. Today, women's ability to access ART allows them to become pregnant and give birth with zero risk of transmitting the virus to their babies. For mothers living with

HIV who want to breastfeed, currently available effective maternal ART has changed everything (see Chapter 4).

Exclusive breastfeeding

The possibility that *exclusive* breastfeeding could be protective against mother-to-child transmission of HIV after birth was first highlighted in research from Durban, South Africa, published in 1999 and 2001.[8,9] Exclusive breastfeeding means that the baby receives only breastmilk. Feeding other foods and liquids (even water) to a baby younger than six months damages the baby's gut, causing inflammation which more easily allows any virus in breastmilk to come into contact with the baby's bloodstream (see Chapter 5). The South African researchers found that exclusively breastfed babies had no greater risk of becoming infected than formula-fed babies, who weren't receiving any breastmilk at all. On the other hand, 'mixed feeding' (breastmilk *and* formula-feeding) posed a much greater risk. It was an intriguing finding. Not only did it show that feeding a baby *all* breastmilk posed a lower risk than feeding *some* breastmilk. It also showed that the time of greatest risk to a baby was birth, not breastfeeding. Six years later, the protective effect of exclusive breastfeeding was confirmed by Dr Peter Iliff and colleagues at the ZVITAMBO project in Zimbabwe.[10] The results showed that even three months of exclusive breastfeeding seemed to be protective against the risk of transmission of the virus. On later testing, and even though the mothers had not received any ART, the babies exclusively breastfed for three months showed a transmission risk of 0% and 1.3% respectively at six months, and 5.3% and 5.6% respectively approximately a year later.

Antiretroviral therapy and exclusive breastfeeding together (ART + EBF)

Several research groups in developing countries began extending antiretroviral therapy to cover the period of breastfeeding, on the grounds that it was unethical to withdraw treatment from mothers once they had given birth, leaving them to die.[11,12] Not surprisingly, they found that the longer mothers received ART, e.g. from the first trimester of pregnancy and during breastfeeding until after weaning (instead of just a few weeks or days before and around the time of birth), the greater the protection.

Looking at the importance of viral load, Carla Chibwesha and colleagues in Zambia found that the duration of the mother's antiretroviral treatment was *the most important* predictor of perinatal HIV transmission.[13] For instance, women who had received Highly Active Antiretroviral Therapy (HAART) for less than four weeks had a five-fold increased risk of HIV transmission. It was most effective when mothers received HAART for at least 13 weeks before the birth of the baby, giving a long enough time for viral levels to fall to undetectable.

Finally, studies published between 2007 and 2022 from East and Central Africa (and one which included India) have shown that early and appropriate ART, combined with exclusive breastfeeding for up to six months (ART+EBF), reduces the risk of transmission of HIV through breastfeeding to between 0–1%. Longer follow-up studies also showed that when the vulnerable young baby enjoys the health advantages of exclusive breastfeeding, reaching six months with an intact and undamaged gut, mixed feeding *after* six months does not pose the same risk.[14-22] (More about this in Chapter 5.)

When ART + EBF seems to fail

Even though the risk of HIV transmission through breastfeeding has been reduced to vanishingly tiny percentages, some health professionals still remain sceptical, often pointing to studies which seem to show that breastfeeding poses an unnecessary risk *even when mothers receive ART*. They reason that in countries where formula-feeding is deemed to be safe, the *benefits* of breastfeeding are negligible.

It's important to take these concerns seriously. It's equally important to subject them to close scrutiny. Why do some studies seem to show a reduced risk of transmission through breastfeeding, and others continue to worry the doctors? When mothers are confronted by doubt and scepticism like this, they can ask their doctors to look more closely at the actual journal articles. In other words, read the fine print!

Sometimes review papers are hazy about which babies of which mothers were included in which study, and how many were lost to follow-up. There can be reviews in which apples are compared with oranges, with predictably strange results. And there can be meta-analyses, where results from many papers are mixed together in mind-numbing complexity, making it difficult to unpack what actually happened, and when.

In some of these studies, the duration of exclusive breastfeeding was very short,[23] or the definition of 'breastfed' or 'formula-fed' was misleading; the babies may have been included in an 'intent to treat' analysis, keeping them in their originally assigned group, when in fact their mothers had changed their feeding method during the course of the study. For example, exclusively breastfed babies may have ended up being bottle-fed but their (higher) HIV-infection rates were counted in the exclusively breastfed group. Or apparently formula-fed babies had once again been breastfed. Physiologically it's very difficult to elect to formula-feed from birth and then to take up breastfeeding weeks later (it can be done, but it's difficult). What's more likely is that these 'breastfed' babies were in fact mixed fed from birth.[24] Some review papers concluding that breastfeeding with HIV is risky, particularly those using poor definitions, include studies that are cited on their own, as well as being included in a review or a meta-analysis, effectively counting them twice, and this can make it more likely that the vote comes down on the side of formula-feeding.

In examining the tiny number of apparent failures with the ART + EBF protocol it's particularly important to look at how 'exclusive breastfeeding' was defined:

- Were other foods and liquids permitted in the definition?
- How long did breastfeeding last?
- Was the mother prescribed a long enough course of ART to achieve an undetectable viral load?

> were her viral levels actually tested?
> was she adherent in taking her meds?

The details of who was included in the research, and what was going to be studied are often in the fine print of the methodology section. Careful scrutiny sometimes reveals:

In breastfeeding

- Lapses in exclusive breastfeeding. Check what else was fed to the baby and how often. A study done in Durban which showed a 4% risk of transmission of HIV even for 'exclusively breastfed' babies included babies who might have also received up to three days of extra water, formula or solid foods. For babies who were actually defined as 'mixed-fed' the risk of transmission was ten-fold for babies who had actually received some solid foods, and double for babies mixed fed with formula as well as breastmilk.[25]
- Some oft-cited studies, like the PROMISE study, are so complex, involving groups of babies from different countries and with such different feeding protocols, that they are very difficult to compare or understand.[21]
- One WHO-funded study published in 2011 with a transmission rate of 5% through breastfeeding implied that mothers had received up-to-date counselling to exclusively breastfeed, but most of the babies had, in fact, been mixed fed according to outdated infant feeding guidance from six years previously.[26]

Maternal antiretroviral treatment or infant prophylaxis?

- Mothers received ART for too short a time, i.e. less than the 13 weeks needed to achieve an undetectable viral load, because they presented late in pregnancy, or their babies were born prematurely.[14]
- Mothers failed to take their ART medications as advised (called *adherence*), either:
    > because they believed they had been cured, or had mental health problems, leading in each case to a rebound in viral load,[17] or

> because they moved away from their treatment centre and missed their drug regimens for several months,[22] or even
> because ART treatment for mothers was seen as only necessary for those whose immune systems were already damaged by HIV (with a low CD4 count) instead of for *all* mothers diagnosed as HIV+, as had happened in some early cohorts or women included in the widely cited PROMISE study.[27]

- Citing a study where only *babies* received antiretroviral prophylaxis during breastfeeding for up to a year, and *mothers received no treatment,* (because researchers considered they were not eligible for it; the study was done in the era before WHO recommended life-long treatment from diagnosis[28]), current BHIVA guidance[29] suggests that 'The risk of transmission in *women on combined antiretroviral therapy* does still increase according to the duration of breastfeeding. Women who wish to breastfeed… should be advised to breastfeed for as short a time as possible.' Clearly this is misleading because the babies, *not the mothers*, were receiving ART.
- Recent moves to down-play the risks of mixed feeding before six months suggest that occasional mixed feeding is not risky if a mother's viral load is suppressed. However, there is scant new research to confirm this hypothesis, except for a Canadian study where premature twins received mixed feeding from 6–12 weeks and while the mother received ART, the twins also received antiretroviral prophylaxis from birth until after weaning.[30]

Undetectable=Untransmittable (U=U) for horizontal transmission

As early as 1999 researchers had accumulated overwhelming evidence to show that it was the number of viral copies of HIV in the blood (called the viral load) which determined whether a mother was likely to transmit HIV to her baby; the higher the viral load, the greater the risk.[31] Early research focused on testing a mother's CD4 count to determine both whether she could receive ART and how infectious she might be to her baby. The early studies only provided ART to a mother when her CD4 count had gone down below a certain level (and her viral load had gone up). It was eventually realised that testing an individual's viral load might be a more effective way to gauge infectivity[32] and that all mothers diagnosed with HIV should receive immediate treatment regardless.

Today, the goal of antiretroviral therapy is viral suppression to an undetectable level – viral load that is so low that it cannot be detected by a viral load test. A high viral load or a viral load blip (over 50 copies/ml) in a mother on treatment indicates:

- either that she has received ART for too short a time
- or that the medication is not being taken properly (she has low adherence)
- or that she is experiencing drug resistance, and her ART may need to be changed[33]

The protective effect of undetectable viral load against infecting another individual was also found to apply to horizontal transmission between sexual partners by researchers working in Uganda as early as 2000.[34]

These remarkable findings led Swiss researchers to issue a position paper in 2008 called the Swiss Statement,[35] confirming that Undetectable=Untransmittable (U=U). However, it took several years and much further research by others for the concept to be accepted.[36] Finally, two extremely large studies published in 2016 and 2019 looking at both heterosexual or homosexual transmission between serodiscordant couples (meaning one is infected and the other is not) showed that transmission doesn't happen when the infected partner receives sufficient ART to maintain an undetectable viral load. Thousands of couples participated without a single infection being recorded.[37, 38]

U=U for vertical transmission during pregnancy and birth

Research reported in 2022 from France confirmed that mothers (who did not breastfeed) on ART from before conception and who continued ART throughout pregnancy, with an undetectable viral load (<50 copies/ml) 'can eliminate perinatal transmission of HIV'.[39]

A similar strategy has been proposed to protect against the risk of vertical transmission through breastfeeding.[40] Pietro Vernazza, who helped to develop the Swiss Statement, has described the 'ideal scenario' that would need to be in place,[41] maintaining that 'we have no evidence of proven transmission' when:

- Mothers receive ART from the first trimester of pregnancy to achieve an undetectable viral load
- Mothers are adherent to their medication
- Babies are exclusively breastfed for the first six months of life

In a large study conducted in Tanzania with extensive follow-up of babies who were breastfed for six months or more,[19] no cases of postnatal transmission occurred for mothers who stayed in the programme, adhered to their ART, and had a suppressed viral load.

Local data

British healthcare providers may be understandably nervous about encouraging breastfeeding in the context of HIV while there is little published research from high-resource countries. They contend that overseas study results cannot be generalised to First World countries. Data has been sparse due in part to the fact that mothers with HIV living in Europe, North America and other resource-rich settings have mostly been advised not to breastfeed, and conducting a prospective randomised controlled trial allocating some babies to breastfeeding and some to formula-feeding would be deemed unethical. As a result, we are left with a Catch-22 situation.

However, we do have data! Since 2006, retrospective statistics on MTCT of HIV in the UK have been collected by an agency under the umbrella of Public Health England, attached to UCL Great Ormond Street Institute of Child Health in London. It has had a few name-changes over the years, but is currently known as the Integrated Screening Outcomes Surveillance Service (ISOSS) and is reputedly the largest register documenting breastfeeding with HIV in the Western world. The register records monthly viral load test results of mothers, as well as monthly HIV test results for the babies, and duration and exclusivity of breastfeeding. A July 2021 *Report* described how, between 2012 and March 2020, 150 babies had been breastfed by mothers with HIV on suppressive viral therapy, for times ranging from one day to two years (with a median time of 3–16 weeks).[42]

As at November 2022, there were no transmissions among infants breastfed when BHIVA guidance was followed.[43]

Data from other high-resource settings

Other researchers have collected data on smaller numbers of babies being breastfed by mothers living with HIV in other countries in North America and Europe:

- *Germany:* At a Comittée des Familles HIV and Breastfeeding Symposium held in Paris in October 2021, researcher Annette Haberle presented data documenting 40 babies breastfed by mothers living with HIV. In 15 treatment centres, the number of women with HIV who breastfed increased over time from zero to two women per year between 2009 and 2016 to nine to 13 women per year between 2017 and 2019.[44] In another study there were no transmissions among 30 women who breastfed with HIV, even though optimal viral suppression was not always achieved. Infant prophylaxis ranged from four weeks of zidovudine (ZDV) to three-drug ARV regimens using therapeutic doses for the duration of breastfeeding.[45]
- *Switzerland:* In Switzerland a further five cases have been reported where clinicians and mothers used shared decision-making to facilitate breastfeeding.[46]

- *Canada:* A group in Toronto described three breastfed infants with no transmission via breastfeeding.[30] However, as noted previously, two of these babies were pre-term twins who received extended triple antiretroviral prophylaxis while being breastfed with formula supplements from 6–12 weeks. Thus the risk of premature mixed feeding was effectively offset by infant PrEP.
- *United States of America:* Three studies record women with HIV breastfeeding in the US: among nine women with 10 pregnancies in Maryland,[47] eight women with HIV breastfed at a second site in Washington DC,[48] and 10 women who breastfed a further 13 infants in Colorado,[49] there were no transmissions. Among 93 US clinicians who provide specialty care to women with HIV, one-third of the providers were aware that women in their care breastfed their infants after being advised not to do so.[50]
- *Italy:* 13 women studied prospectively had no transmissions of HIV through breastfeeding.[51]
- *Belgium:* two cases of HIV+ women who wanted to breastfeed were supported, and their babies were not infected.[52]

International guidelines on HIV and infant feeding

Appreciation of the competing risks of breastfeeding vs formula-feeding for child survival led to formulation of new international recommendations in 2009. These were further refined in 2016 to recommend that mothers living with HIV should receive ART from diagnosis, to be continued for life, and that breastfeeding should once again be supported.[53]

UK national HIV and infant feeding recommendations

Successful interventions in the UK have brought the chance of a baby being born with HIV almost to vanishing point. Women are tested during early pregnancy, and are able to receive ART well in time to achieve an undetectable viral load by their estimated date of delivery.

In 2009, the British HIV Association held a public consultation on HIV and infant feeding. It was acknowledged that while mothers with HIV in the UK should be advised to formula-feed, individual mothers might really want to breastfeed, and their choice should be supported. Current British HIV Association guidelines for the management of HIV in pregnancy and postpartum[29] give the following carefully drafted advice, which begins with recommending formula-feeding, but then concedes that women who choose to breastfeed should be supported to do so with extra monitoring:

> *In the UK and other high-income settings, the safest way to feed infants born to women with HIV is with formula milk, as there is on-going risk of HIV exposure after birth. We therefore continue to recommend that women living with HIV feed their babies with formula milk...*

> *Women who are virologically suppressed on combination ART with good adherence and who choose to breastfeed should be supported to do so, but should be informed about the low risk of transmission of HIV through breastfeeding in this situation and the requirement for extra maternal and infant clinical monitoring.*

This guidance simultaneously provides information to enable clinicians to comply with current recommendations, and at the same time offers them a way to support HIV+ mothers who want to breastfeed. This would seem to constitute a win-win situation – protection for the clinician, and support for the mother. In my experience this is exactly what happens – mothers are advised by the major support groups and agencies that formula-feeding is recommended, but if they make their wishes to breastfeed clear, then their healthcare providers are often extremely helpful in supporting their goals while monitoring mother and baby's health and well-being.

US HIV and infant feeding recommendations

In January 2013, the American Academy of Pediatrics (AAP)

published revised guidance on HIV and infant feeding[54] to allow that an HIV-infected woman receiving effective antiretroviral therapy with repeatedly undetectable HIV viral loads may choose to breastfeed. The AAP recommended that a pediatric expert should be consulted on how to minimise postpartum transmission risk including:

- exclusive breastfeeding
- careful monitoring of maternal viral load
- adherence to maternal ART
- prompt administration of antimicrobial agents in instances of clinical mastitis
- monitoring of infant HIV infection status throughout lactation and at 4–6 weeks and 3–6 months after weaning

Recently, organisations supporting women living with HIV in the US have succeeded in opening a dialogue with policy-makers on the matter of breastfeeding with HIV.[55] On 31 January 2023, the US Panel on Treatment of HIV in Pregnancy and Prevention of Perinatal Transmission and the Panel on Antiretroviral Therapy and Medical Management of Children Living with HIV[56] issued recommendations that clinicians engage parents in *patient-centered counseling and shared decision-making* regarding infant feeding. The updated guidance on Infant Feeding for Individuals with HIV in the United States, published by ClinicalInfo at the end of January 2023, clarifies:

- *Replacement feeding with formula or banked pasteurized donor human milk is recommended to eliminate the risk of HIV transmission through breastfeeding when people with HIV are not on ART and/or do not have a suppressed viral load during pregnancy (at a minimum throughout the third trimester), as well as at delivery.*
- *Individuals with HIV who are on ART with a sustained undetectable viral load and who choose to breastfeed should be supported in this decision.*
- *Engaging Child Protective Services or similar agencies is not an appropriate response to the infant feeding choices of an individual with HIV.*

- *Clinicians are encouraged to consult the national Perinatal HIV/ AIDS hotline (1-888-448-8765) with questions about infant feeding by individuals with HIV.*

Other First World countries

Following the British model Australia (NAPWHA)[57] and New Zealand (NZ Ministry of Health)[58] have relaxed their absolute prohibition on breastfeeding with HIV. They recommend formula-feeding but permit breastfeeding, and urge mothers to fully discuss their wishes with their healthcare providers.

Shared decision-making

Ultimately, by far the best course is to discuss your wishes with your HIV clinicians and your healthcare team in the light of current research and your own health, so that you can receive your doctor's tailor-made medical advice and full support which is specific to *your unique circumstances*. While your doctor provides medical advice and information, the final decision about how to feed your baby is yours. It helps to remember that everyone wants the best for your baby. More information on this is provided in Chapter 3.

3. ADVANCE PLANNING AND ENLISTING HELP

Women living with HIV who are considering breastfeeding usually begin searching for as much information as they can find about the risks and benefits of breastfeeding vs formula-feeding quite early on in their pregnancies (see Chapter 2). Some have dreamed of being able to breastfeed even before they become pregnant. Having the needed conversations about your goals with your HIV clinicians and doctors helps you to plan wisely.

Starting in 2010, and up to the present time, the British HIV Association (BHIVA) guidance has been clear that their first recommendation is that mothers living with HIV in the UK should formula-feed their babies.[1] However BHIVA accept that *'not breastfeeding can come at an emotional, financial and social cost to women living with HIV'*, and they advise that women receive appropriate support from their HIV multidisciplinary team (which may include peer support, psychological and practical support, and financial support for formula-feeding). They also say that:

> *'Women who are virologically suppressed on cART with good adherence and who choose to breastfeed should be supported to do so, but should be informed about the low risk of transmission of HIV through breastfeeding.'*

Early in 2023, the US Panel on Treatment of HIV in Pregnancy and Prevention of Perinatal Transmission and the Panel on Antiretroviral Therapy and Medical Management of Children Living with HIV issued updated recommendations that clinicians engage parents in *patient-centered counseling and shared decision-making* regarding infant feeding.[2]

Including key people in your discussions

As you make the decision to breastfeed, and carry out your plans in the following weeks or months, you may want to include the other important people in your life. The baby's father, your family, and of course your doctors and medical advisors will be your main sources of information, and emotional and practical support.

It's vitally important that you discuss your wish to breastfeed with your own healthcare providers, so that:

- your goals are known
- your and your baby's special healthcare needs are taken into consideration
- you can receive professional specialist medical advice from your doctors, who know you best
- the best outcome can be reached, taking into consideration both the risks and benefits of breastfeeding for you and your baby, as well as the risks and benefits of *not* breastfeeding for you both.

Making an informed choice

To be able to make an informed choice about whether you want to breastfeed, you will need to discuss with your HIV clinician:

- why you want to breastfeed
- current information and research on HIV and breastfeeding (see chapters 1, 2, 4 and 5)
- the risks and benefits of breastfeeding generally
- current national policy recommendations
- your viral load, and your health history
- how your baby's health will be monitored

Your HIV clinician

Mothers living with HIV who have chosen to breastfeed usually start by booking a long appointment with their HIV clinician. Fully discussing your goals, and the implications of the research on HIV and breastfeeding with a specialist (see Chapter 2), means that you can go through every aspect of what your choice will mean. Mothers often describe the exceptional response and very positive reactions they receive from their HIV specialists, for example a prenatal consultation lasting two hours or more in which the mother was able to fully discuss the research she had heard about, and find out the implications for her particular situation.

Your history and plans

Your doctors will be reassured by knowing that you:

- have a fully suppressed viral load at least during the last trimester of pregnancy, and preferably since early pregnancy or even before conception
- have a good history of adhering meticulously to your ART
- have been regularly attending your HIV clinic appointments and check-ups
- are happy to attend a monthly clinic review
- accept that your baby will receive infant antiretroviral prophylaxis for several weeks to protect against viral transfer at birth
- will agree to monthly testing:
    > of your viral load
    > of your baby's HIV status

A team approach

Breastfeeding with HIV straddles several disciplines. Ideally your care will be coordinated and facilitated in a multi-disciplinary team approach. Your lactation consultant or breastfeeding counsellor should make herself available to liaise with and be guided by your doctors, midwives and hospital staff as everyone works towards achieving the best outcome for you and your baby.

You will receive care from many different professionals as you navigate your infant-feeding choices and make all the practical arrangements. Once your pregnancy is confirmed you will need referrals from your HIV clinician to all the members of the team (mentioned below) who will be caring for you and your baby. Ascertain from your HIV clinician that they are able to act as a resource for the other doctors and staff who will be looking after you during your pregnancy, around the time of birth, and afterwards. Ideally they will be able to liaise with other members of the team, and act as your advocate, communicating your wish to breastfeed to all the professionals who will be caring for you and your baby.

Your healthcare providers and their experience of breastfeeding

Healthcare providers may be aware of the current policy endorsement that mothers living with HIV should be supported in their choice to breastfeed. However, in practice, they may never have worked with a mother who has this ambition. Some doctors will take the time and trouble to contact colleagues who may have previously worked with other mothers with HIV to help them breastfeed with a view to exchanging information and providing professional support.

ISOSS surveillance and reporting to the Enhanced Register

Additionally, your healthcare providers may wish to know about the Integrated Screening Outcomes Surveillance Service, previously known as the National Surveillance of HIV in Pregnancy and Childhood.[3] This organisation compiles data on women with HIV and their breastfed babies in an Enhanced Register so that the information will contribute to epidemiological data for the future.[4] Mothers can request that their healthcare providers access the ISOSS information. Your own baby's HIV status, and whether or not you breastfeed, will also be monitored by ISOSS.

In the US, clinicians who are caring for a mother with HIV who is considering breastfeeding should consult with an expert and feel free to call the National Perinatal HIV Hotline (1-888-448-8765 or nccc.ucsf.edu/clinician-consultation/perinatal-hiv-aids).

Make a breastfeeding plan

Once you have decided with your clinician whether breastfeeding is a good choice for you and your baby, it is time to think about clearly communicating your wishes to the rest of your team. Mothers living with HIV who succeeded in breastfeeding have described how helpful it has been to have a breastfeeding plan as an extension of your birth plan.

So that everyone is confident about supporting your wish to breastfeed, right from the beginning, your breastfeeding plan should be signed off by all the members of your healthcare team:

- your HIV clinician
- your obstetrician
- your baby's paediatrician (you may need an advance appointment to discuss your feeding choice)
- the maternity unit/midwives/doulas/hospital staff where your baby will be born
- your community nurse/health visitor/postnatal health clinic, who will be checking on your baby's well-being in the months that you will be breastfeeding
- your general practitioner and doctor's surgery
- any other health professional who will have the care of you or your baby
- your lactation consultant or breastfeeding counsellor

Your breastfeeding plan should allow for special care in the scenarios set out below. It should cover your wish for help in the specific areas where breastfeeding with HIV may differ from breastfeeding outside the context of HIV, for example:

- no routine oral suctioning after birth (in order not to damage the baby's mouth or throat).
- uninterrupted skin-to-skin contact with your baby after birth to facilitate early breastfeeding, and delay any non-urgent procedures until after the first breastfeed.

- no mother-baby separation for routine medical protocols, e.g. the first bath, blood tests etc. If these are required, they should be carried out at the bedside.
- if the baby requires any medical tests or procedures which require him/her to be taken to another part of the hospital, then you, or the baby's father, or another trusted person will be permitted to accompany him at all times.
- no supplements for your baby (nothing except your milk) unless they are medically indicated/prescribed, and the need for them fully discussed with you, including sugar water, glucose solution, infant formula, colic remedies, vitamin supplements, extra waters/teas and traditional foods (see Chapter 13).
- help to position and attach your baby to the breast within 1–2 hours of birth if possible, and continued help and follow-up while you and the baby learn how to breastfeed.
- delay hospital discharge until the baby is breastfeeding well.
- assistance with learning how to hand-express breastmilk and spoon-feeding expressed breastmilk if there is a latching difficulty, pending acquiring breastfeeding skills.
- no medications unless they are prescribed.
- no frenotomy i.e. surgical division of the lingual frenulum (tie under the baby's tongue) or of the labial or buccal frenula (ties under the lips or cheeks), sometimes recommended to help a baby to latch more easily to the breast, to facilitate breastfeeding efficiency or to reduce mother's nipple pain and trauma. If, in the unlikely event that your breastfeeding specialist cannot resolve these difficulties with other strategies and believes *that there is no other remedy*, then breastfeeding direct should be suspended until healing has taken place.
- prompt care from your general practitioner, and advice about the need for antibiotics should you show symptoms of mastitis (see Chapter 12).
- where and when monthly HIV viral load tests for you and HIV testing for your baby will be carried out, and how soon you'll be able to receive the results. Be sure to receive clarity on this aspect.

- the baby to be weighed on the day of birth, at three days and, if breastfeeding is going well, weekly thereafter for the first six weeks, then fortnightly, and then monthly up to six months.
- solid/weaning foods should not be started before six months.

Antiretroviral prophylaxis for the baby

In the UK the pregnant mother who has HIV will have received ART for many months (and sometimes years) before her baby's due date and this is ideal so that she can achieve an undetectable viral load by the time the baby is born. After birth, babies may receive 2–6 weeks of ARV prophylaxis after birth (BHIVA recommends 2–4 weeks depending on the mother's viral load,[5] WHO recommends 4–6 weeks), to protect against viral exposure during labour and birth (not breastfeeding).

In the UK, ART for the mother is the preferred treatment rather than continued infant prophylaxis.[1] In the US breastfed babies of mothers living with HIV may receive ARV prophylaxis for times varying from 4–6 weeks to the whole duration of breastfeeding depending on the protocols of individual HIV specialists.[2] Despite the lack of data to support treating both the mother and infant during breastfeeding, some experts feel more comfortable continuing infant ARV prophylaxis (using nevirapine) during breastfeeding and for 1–4 weeks after weaning, even when the mother is receiving suppressive ART.[6]

Testing and monitoring

For mothers who are breastfeeding, current BHIVA and ClinicalInfo guidance recommends monthly testing of the mother's viral load, and of the baby's HIV status. You can expect:

HIV tests for the baby:

- Within 48 hours after birth
- At two weeks
- Monthly for the duration of breastfeeding
- At four and eight weeks after the end of breastfeeding

- Antibody testing at 22–24 months or eight weeks after stopping breastfeeding, whichever is the later.

Testing and monitoring may be characterised as inconvenient, either for you or for your healthcare providers, but it can be reassuring to know that you and your baby are doing well. Most mothers feel relieved and happy to receive their own and their baby's bloodwork results every month, and to know that breastfeeding continues to be safe and their babies remain healthy.

During Covid-19 lockdowns BHIVA discouraged breastfeeding because of the anticipated difficulty in mothers and babies receiving their viral load and HIV tests.[7] However, mothers who did not know of this ruling continued to attend their clinic appointments and receive blood tests as usual and didn't experience any difficulty. Nevertheless, it may be worth discussing in advance what arrangements will be made for you and your baby to receive recommended monitoring.

Additional checks and balances

There can be other lab work and testing which may be helpful too.

- One HIV clinician in a regional hospital made arrangements with colleagues in advance that if there was any concern about whether the mother was having any viral blips, viral testing of her breastmilk could be done by a lab in London. It turned out that this precaution was not necessary after all, but the mother was greatly reassured that the arrangement was set up in advance in case it was needed.
- Should a mother experience mastitis or ongoing sore nipples, milk samples or nipple swabs can be analysed for a bacterial infection. If an infection is found, the lab is able to suggest which antibiotic would be most suitable to treat it, i.e. whether the organism is sensitive or resistant to particular medications. This means that, should it be necessary, appropriate treatment can be started without delay, saving pain and discomfort as well

as limiting the amount of time that direct breastfeeding might need to be temporarily suspended (see chapters 12 and 13).
- Regular infant weight monitoring can reassure a mother, or indeed a health worker, that exclusive breastfeeding is adequate for a demanding baby, i.e. that the mother is making enough milk. Evidence of good weekly gains, particularly in the first 2–3 months, can demonstrate to an anxious mother or a concerned health visitor that the baby is thriving on mother's milk alone. If the baby gains less than expected, there is an early warning that something needs to change so that he gets a bit more milk (see Chapter 14 for more info). If the weight gain is good it can boost a mother's confidence that her milk is all her baby needs to grow and thrive.

Help with breastfeeding

Contrary to popular belief, breastfeeding is not 'natural' and instinctive. It is, in fact, a learned behaviour. The best way to learn is by having watched young babies being breastfed by other family members, aunties, sisters or close friends. But in the UK, with its low breastfeeding rates, you may not have had the opportunity to closely observe very small babies at the breast. So you may want to seek outside help.

It will be worthwhile learning as much as you can about breastfeeding before your baby is born. Can you attend antenatal breastfeeding preparation classes? Can you find a breastfeeding mother-support group where you can observe other mothers and babies of all ages and hear about the normal challenges and successes that happen during normal breastfeeding?

Finding a breastfeeding specialist that you know you can call on any time after your baby arrives is also a wise plan. Babies don't have weekends or holidays, so you will want to find someone who is available 24/7, who might offer home visits or online consultations should you need them, and of course someone who has a clear knowledge of the special needs of breastfeeding in the context of HIV.

A comparison of training, experience and qualifications of various types of breastfeeding practitioners has been compiled by Lactation Consultants of Great Britain.[8] Different kinds of help are out there, and it may be worth doing your homework to find out who is likely to be the best fit for you. Sources of assistance could include:

- A private practice International Board Certified Lactation Consultant (IBCLC).[9]
- A breastfeeding counsellor from one of the main support groups, who can be found through the UK National Breastfeeding Helpline.[10]
- Breastfeeding support group meetings, offered by organisations such as La Leche League, the Breastfeeding Network, the Academy of Breastfeeding Medicine or National Childbirth Trust. See the GP Infant Support Network info.[11]
- General breastfeeding information written for mothers, available in books and written material published by or endorsed by the main breastfeeding support groups.
- Your midwife, GP, health visitor or the NHS Breastfeeding Support Service for help in your postcode.[12] Be sure to ask if they have had special training in lactation and breastfeeding.

Hospital discharge

It's a good idea to stay in the hospital until your baby is latching and breastfeeding well, so that you can access practical help should you need it. Having the hospital midwives or the hospital lactation consultant show you how to latch your baby to the breast should be part of your routine care. Alternatively, if you're not confident by the time you go home, it's advisable to see a private practice IBCLC who can make a home visit and fine-tune your latching techniques. In the meantime, ensure that you ask for help to learn how to express or pump your milk, and feed it to the baby by cup, spoon, or bottle while he learns what to do. (See Chapter 10 for expressing/pumping/storing breastmilk, and Chapter 13 for feeding the baby expressed breastmilk).

Breast pumps

For a mother living with HIV who needs to ensure that she has a good milk supply, which means good breast care to prevent damage to her milk-producing cells (see Chapter 12), having a good, effective, hospital-grade double electric breast pump can save the day. If breastfeeding gets off to an excellent start and you have a baby who knows how to breastfeed straight away, you may never need a pump. And you may not need a pump for very long, whatever happens, so you don't necessarily need to go to the expense of buying one, but knowing where you can access a pump if you need one is good insurance. Some organisations will hire out pumps on 24 hours' notice. An internet search will usually provide more information about costs, providers and tips.[13] It's a good idea to arrange access to a pump in advance, so that you can head off breast over-fullness in the first few days after birth. Once it's happened it becomes an emergency and in the context of HIV it's imperative to resolve engorgement promptly, and ideally to avoid it. The small rental fee may be well worth the investment.

Planning in advance for when and how you will stop breastfeeding

The normal course of breastfeeding has been shown to last anywhere from 2–7 years.[14] If there is any possibility that you'll want to wean at six months, or before the baby himself shows that he no longer wants to breastfeed, it will be easier to do so if your baby is already familiar with occasional bottle-feeding or using a dummy for comfort. Keep this in mind as you and your baby become more and more reliant on breastfeeding for comfort as well as food.

Additional HIV and breastfeeding information

Some mothers keep a folder of papers, plans, research articles and breastfeeding information that they can refer to as necessary. They may also share and discuss these resources with their doctors, midwives or health visitors. The information in this book is not intended to replace medical advice, and mothers should fully discuss any of the suggestions with their healthcare team, to be sure that it is relevant and safe for them and their babies.

To begin with, some healthcare staff may be a little dubious and doubtful, but then develop an interest in this special situation, and may want to read your materials for themselves, so keep them handy! One mother was delighted to be asked to help her doctor prepare written guidance for breastfeeding with HIV to help educate his junior doctors. Another mother was recruited into focus group discussions intended to provide background information for a study on attitudes towards breastfeeding by mothers living with HIV.

It's a good idea to enlist the help of an experienced lactation consultant or breastfeeding counsellor in case you and your baby would benefit from assistance with latching your baby to the breast, with breast care, or with special information on breastfeeding with HIV. Ensure that you pick someone you feel you can trust with your history, and who is knowledgeable and experienced on the subject of HIV and breastfeeding – or can find out for you.

Filtering out irrelevant breastfeeding information

If you decide to breastfeed, you'll find that family and friends won't hesitate to share their experiences with you. It's helpful if your support network, including health professionals or a lactation consultant, is aware of your HIV status, so that the help and information they offer can take into account knowledge of safely breastfeeding with HIV.

If your support people don't know your HIV status, you may receive inappropriate information. One mother who had sore nipples was pestered repeatedly by a health visitor who strongly recommended that her baby undergo a frenotomy for a mild tongue tie,[15] even going so far as to make an urgent appointment for the baby to have the procedure done as an emergency. Clearly the health visitor did not know that this would be risky for an HIV-exposed breastfed baby. (The baby went on to breastfeed without incident, with an intact frenulum.)

Similarly, family, friends or professionals may suggest formula supplements (either to give you a break, or if they think that the baby is not thriving), not knowing that mixed feeding under six months is a risk for your baby. People usually mean well, but to make it really relevant to your unique situation, you can either disclose your status to key people, or filter the information you receive.

Disclosure

In general, women are strongly encouraged to inform partners and close family members, and healthcare providers (including midwives, health visitors and GPs), and anyone else involved in their care (such as lactation consultants), about their HIV status. This enables the family and the healthcare team to give appropriate support and advice, especially regarding feeding, vaccinations and medical assessment of the baby. However, mothers living with HIV are understandably cautious about revealing their HIV status too widely. They fear ostracism and stigma if people know that they have HIV. You are entitled to maintain confidentiality about your HIV status and you will want to think carefully about who you disclose it to. While there will be some people who don't need to know, there will be others who can provide you with better care and assistance if they do know about your positive status. There will be others still who, by being kept in the dark, may provide you with inappropriate information – you'll need to keep this possibility in mind.

Retaining legal counsel

The prime reason for talking over your wishes with your HIV clinical team is so that you can all work together for the best outcome for you and your baby. While it is clear that blanket prohibitions against breastfeeding with HIV are no longer seen as acceptable anywhere, even in most First World countries, it is always worthwhile finding out well in advance what the HIV and infant feeding policy guidelines are in your local area.

Sometimes updated recommendations on breastfeeding with

HIV are slow to be adopted by individual hospital administrators and individual doctors. It has happened that staff who know and support your decisions may not be on duty, or new, less knowledgeable staff may prioritise formula-feeding over breastfeeding. Breastfeeding with HIV may be viewed as a safeguarding issue – as some may wrongly worry that it may place your baby at unnecessary risk. A mother living with HIV will very occasionally report that she has been threatened with referral to child protective services or social services if she persists in her wish for a vaginal birth or to breastfeed her baby.

If there is any possibility at all that this could happen to you, it may give you peace of mind to retain a solicitor or attorney well in advance to provide legal protection and speak for you. I have, in the past, found lawyers who are willing to make arrangements in advance of the birth, in order to make a hospital visit at a moment's notice should this happen. Having a retainer agreement that you have arranged in advance guarantees you availability and access to legal representation. Bear in mind that you may need to pay a retainer fee, and hopefully you will end up paying for protection that you don't need, but you may well consider that it's worth it. Look on the internet or phone around to find a lawyer/solicitor/ attorney who is knowledgeable about family law and custody issues, tell them your circumstances and ask if they can be available to make a hospital visit at your maternity unit if necessary. There is much peace of mind knowing that your corner will be defended against intimidation of this nature should you need it.

Finally, in extreme circumstances where she has no help, a mother may well decide to comply with bottle-feeding recommendations while in hospital and/or until she can receive clarification so that she can initiate breastfeeding once she gets home (See Transitioning back to breastfeeding in Chapter 14 for how this can be achieved).

Planning your life to accommodate a new baby

Becoming a mother is one of the high points of a woman's life. But everyone agrees that being the mother of a newborn can also be exhausting. If you're able to arrange your life so that you can receive help and support for several weeks after you come home from the hospital, you might find that this is a good investment in getting breastfeeding off to a good start. New mothers usually find that they can easily meet the needs of the new baby – it's the other duties and responsibilities which can feel overwhelming. You might consider:

- setting up a foolproof memory-jogger system so you don't forget to take your ART; new mothers often don't get enough sleep, which can make you forgetful. Taking your ART is crucial for you and for your baby
- enlisting help with housework and meals from your mother, or another trusted friend or relation; you may need someone to 'mother the mother'
- arranging paid help with housework and cleaning, laundry, meal preparation, or childcare for an older toddler
- help with the school run if you have an older child
- dog-walking if you have a pet
- preparing pre-cooked meals
- hiring a doula
- arranging online shopping and home deliveries
- planning for social events well in advance; for example some mothers buy gifts and pre-address birthday and anniversary cards, and even arrange dental and other medical appointments before the birth
- negotiating with your partner what responsibilities he will be able to take over, and for as long as possible, so that you're able to rest and concentrate on breastfeeding your baby
- arranging your day so that you are able to sit and cluster-feed your baby on and off for several hours in the late afternoon and evening (e.g. cook your evening meal in advance, or get in ready-meals or have someone else cook for you). In the first three months, your baby may need to marathon feed between the hours of 4pm and 10pm, and having no other commitments

during these hours will make mothering your baby so much easier and be a very good investment for the future.

A note about visitors who want to come and admire and cuddle your new baby: breastfeeding has been known to falter in the first week because visitors feel they must give the mother a break from the baby, or want to relieve her of baby-care by stretching out the intervals between breastfeeds, so that she can rest. This is not helpful. Certainly accept offers from friends and family to come and see you for a brief visit, but be sure to invite them to make the tea, help with household chores, or play with your older children, leaving you, the mother, to care for and breastfeed your baby. Don't let them stay so long that you become exhausted.

4. THE TRANSFORMATIONAL EFFECT OF ANTIRETROVIRAL THERAPY

Every year in the UK, up to 1,000 mothers living with HIV become pregnant. Current strategies to prevent mother-to-child transmission of the virus have been an unqualified success.[1] If a mother doesn't already know her HIV status, testing in early pregnancy ensures that if she tests positive, she can begin prompt treatment with antiretroviral therapy (ART) to reduce her viral load to undetectable by the time the baby is born and breastfeeding begins. Current guidelines recommend formula-feeding, but concede that if a mother wants to breastfeed, then she should be supported to do so. Finally, her viral load and the baby's HIV status can be tested monthly so that she receives every help to have a healthy baby and to protect her own health.

The importance of maternal antiretroviral therapy

Antiretroviral drugs have changed HIV from a lethal disease, which brought immune destruction, illness and death in its wake, to a chronic, treatable condition, like diabetes. In the context of reducing vertical transmission of HIV through breastfeeding, ART has been described as 'transformational'.[2]

Before antiretroviral treatment for HIV became available, the situation was very different. In 1990, almost half of the babies of HIV-infected mothers became infected themselves, either in the womb, during labour or birth, or during breastfeeding. Infected babies went on to suffer from the progressive destruction of the immune system known as Acquired Immune Deficiency Syndrome (AIDS). One-third died by their first birthday, half before their second birthday, and three-quarters before they were five years old.[3]

Beginning in 1994, the first antiretroviral drugs reduced mother-to-child transmission of HIV (MTCT) by about half when mothers didn't breastfeed and ART became the standard of care in resource-rich settings.[4] Mothers in developing countries usually only received treatment if their immune system was already depleted (as shown by a low CD4 cell count), and only then for a few weeks in late pregnancy and during labour. Treatment was stopped once the baby was born. Mothers' milk began to be viewed as a major cause of HIV infection; it was seen as wasteful for mothers to receive ART to 'save' babies from transmission of the virus during pregnancy or birth, only to see them become infected afterwards through breastfeeding.[5]

Today, the recommendation is that all women who receive a positive diagnosis of HIV should take ART immediately and for life. When she receives and takes her medication for at least the last trimester of her pregnancy, a mother can reduce the amount of virus in her blood and in her milk to levels which are virtually undetectable on current HIV tests.[6] A low or undetectable viral load not only keeps the mother healthy so that she can enjoy a normal lifespan, but also reduces the risk of her baby becoming infected by any route to almost nil.

ART adherence is critically important

It is important that you continue your ART to maintain a viral load of <50 copies/ml. There is some research which suggests that new mothers may not always take their drugs. This is not my experience: the mothers I have worked with have been completely committed to adhering to their ART regimens, not just because the drugs help them maintain an undetectable viral load for breastfeeding, but also because they are keen to maintain their own best health so that they can look after their children as they grow up.

Antiretroviral prophylaxis

In the UK your baby will be given post-exposure prophylaxis (PEP) within four hours of delivery, which will usually be continued for 2–4 weeks depending on the mother's viral load.[7,8] BHIVA advise that a baseline venous blood test should be taken on day 1. If the baby were to receive a positive test result then he should be referred immediately for treatment. An already-infected baby benefits from being breastfed since the immunological components of mother's milk help to protect him from other infections.[9] The baby can usually be discharged home once medical and nursing staff are happy that he is tolerating his oral antiretroviral medication. It is important for the baby to receive his prophylaxis and you should seek help if he doesn't tolerate it, or if he becomes unwell at all.

In the USA many clinicians have usually recommended that ART prophylaxis extend for the full period of breastfeeding.[10] However, ClinicalInfo recommendations for antiretroviral prophylaxis for the breastfed baby were revised at the end of January 2023.[11] A consensus on the duration of infant ART for newborns could not be reached. Most members of the policy-making panel agreed to adopt the BHIVA recommendation of only two weeks' prophylaxis; others prefer 4–6 weeks; still others prefer to follow the WHO recommendation for six weeks' ART for infants at low risk of HIV transmission, and some continue to opt for dosing throughout the breastfeeding period. Infant antiretroviral prophylaxis has also been used for the breastfed baby to offset the risk of transmission of HIV during mixed feeding before six months[12] and when the mother has had a viral blip.[13] Your breastfed baby will receive HIV RNA PCR testing at two weeks, six weeks, three months, several weeks after weaning from the breast, and a final antibody test at 22–24 months. Mothers find these tests reassuring to confirm that their baby remains healthy.

Breastfeeding recommendations

After research had revealed that when mothers received ART during pregnancy breastfeeding transmission of HIV could be reduced to extremely low rates, WHO acknowledged in 2009 that higher rates of HIV-free survival could only be achieved by reversing former recommendations for replacement feeding to once again promote breastfeeding. In the same year, the British HIV Association held a public consultation on HIV and infant feeding and tailored their guidance to reflect the aspirations of mothers living with HIV in the UK.

Guidance on HIV and infant feeding varies from country to country, and ranges from a clear prohibition of breastfeeding in countries such as France, to a concession in the UK, the USA and New Zealand that some mothers with HIV might want to breastfeed and their wishes should be supported.

ART + EBF, the ideal combination

Research has shown that the risk of mother-to-child transmission of HIV through breastfeeding is virtually ZERO when a mother living with HIV:

- receives ART early in pregnancy, and for life
- is adherent to her ART and
- exclusively breastfeeds her baby for the first six months of life

The importance of exclusive breastfeeding and why it is protective against HIV is set out in Chapter 5.

5. WHY EXCLUSIVE BREASTFEEDING MATTERS

As we know, breastfeeding is an unequalled way of providing ideal food for the healthy growth and development of infants; it also has important implications for the health of mothers such as reduced risk of breast and ovarian cancers, improved heart health, and a reduced risk of diabetes and osteoporosis in later life.[1]

Just as exclusive breastfeeding for babies (vs mixed breastfeeding before six months) is protective against any disease,[2] so mothers with HIV who choose to breastfeed also need to know that exclusive breastfeeding for the first six months of life is protective against HIV transmission (see Chapter 2). Exclusive breastfeeding means giving the baby no other foods or liquids at all, not even a sip of water. This in turn means that new mothers with HIV, and those advising them, need to take a little extra care to ensure that they know how to bring in an excellent breastmilk supply, sufficient to feed their babies nothing but their own milk for six full months. Mothers can learn self-care techniques to manage their own lactation and how to recognise and resolve small problems in the most efficient, safe way and before they escalate. Should supplements really be necessary, they need to be aware of a safe way to manage combined breast and formula-feeding in the context of HIV, and how they can return to exclusive breastfeeding when the problem is resolved (see Chapter 14). These things *can* be done.

Current universal breastfeeding recommendations

The World Health Organization (WHO) and the American Academy of Paediatrics recommend that infants should be exclusively breastfed with no other foods or liquids besides breastmilk, until six months of age.[3,4]

Exclusive breastfeeding is not common

When mothers receive the right information at the right time they can ensure they have plenty of milk to exclusively breastfeed for the first six months. However, even though most of the world's babies are breastfed, and even where breastfeeding is universal and prolonged, less than half of them receive nothing but their mother's milk for the recommended six months. While formula-feeding is rare in developing countries, babies are traditionally given little sips of water, or little mouthfuls of porridge, from an early age. In First World countries, formula-feeding is often seen as more usual and more convenient than breastfeeding. In the UK we have almost the lowest breastfeeding rates in the world. When healthcare providers receive little training in breastfeeding and may not have breastfed their own babies, they have little experience to offer to new mothers. The last Infant Feeding Survey in 2010 found that three-quarters of British babies had already received formula by 40 days of age, only 34% of babies were receiving any breastmilk by six months and only one in 100 (1%) were fed according to global recommendations.[5] Because breastfeeding has been actively discouraged, few local doctors and HIV clinicians have actually worked with mothers living with HIV who want to breastfeed.

Will my baby receive enough calories and fluids if he receives nothing but my milk?

Outside breastfeeding support circles, there has always been scepticism about whether mother's milk alone will provide enough nutrition and enough water to keep a baby healthy, yet there is a whole body of literature showing that babies thrive on breastmilk alone.[6] Current weight charts developed by WHO, compiled from research in six countries on exclusively breastfed babies, show how healthy babies grow when they are breastfed on demand by healthy mothers.[7] Because extra foods or fluids displace breastmilk and don't increase calorie intake, but do increase the risk of gastroenteritis, exclusively breastfed babies suffer fewer infections.[8]

Since breastmilk is 88% water and contains just the right balance of electrolytes to keep a baby well hydrated, breastfed babies don't need extra water, even in hot climates.[9,10] Babies who are thirsty will want to breastfeed more often and should be trusted to know what they need. It took until 2001 for WHO to issue a formal recommendation that babies should be exclusively breastfed for the first half-year of life[11] and doubts still persist. Even today, mothers will receive inappropriate advice to start solid foods at four months instead of six. For the baby possibly exposed to HIV this is risky because of the immaturity of the baby's gut.

Exclusive vs mixed breastfeeding in the context of HIV

Although, as shown above, the advantages of exclusive breastfeeding compared to partial breastfeeding have been known for decades,[12] most of the world's HIV-exposed breastfed babies were still traditionally supplemented with other foods and liquids at an early age. Anna Coutsoudis in South Africa was the first researcher to apply the known benefits of exclusive breastfeeding to research on the risk of transmission of HIV through breastfeeding,[13] two years before the WHO recommendations endorsed it for all babies and 10 years before HIV and infant feeding guidelines were amended to once more support breastfeeding. Professor Coutsoudis hypothesised that mother's milk contains growth factors which help the baby's gut to mature, while at the same time breastmilk alone would help to maintain gut integrity and so help protect against transmission of HIV. The intestinal epithelial barrier is one of the largest interfaces between the environment and the baby's body. It limits the passage of harmful antigens and microorganisms into the body, and assures the absorption of nutrients and water. The South African researchers found that there was no increased risk of HIV transmission when babies were exclusively breastfed for the first three months of life compared to babies who were exclusively formula-fed. And compared to mixed-fed babies, there was a much lower risk of transmission (14.6% vs 24.1%). In 2001 the same group of researchers published a follow-up paper[14] showing that the protective effect of exclusive breastfeeding against HIV lasted even beyond its duration. By 15 months, the cumulative probability of transmission remained lower among those babies who had been exclusively breastfed for three months than among those who had been mixed fed.

This finding did nothing to change the HIV and infant feeding guidelines in place at the time because WHO were not willing to rely on the results of only one study. The protective effect of exclusive breastfeeding in the context of HIV was not confirmed until 2005. The very large and prestigious ZVITAMBO project in Zimbabwe[15] provided very careful support to mothers to exclusively breastfeed, and found that HIV-transmission that could be attributable to breastfeeding was only 1.3% in the first three months. Even feeding the infant with water and other non-milk liquids increased the risk. Mixed feeding increased the risk four-fold. Early exclusive breastfeeding achieved a 75% reduction in transmission in babies tested at six months.

Finally, these studies were followed by another from Gerry Coovadia and colleagues in Durban in 2007.[16] Their research was designed to assess HIV transmission risks associated with exclusive breastfeeding compared with other types of infant feeding. The key finding was that early introduction of solid foods and animal milks *increased* HIV transmission compared with exclusive breastfeeding from birth. Unfortunately, as previously mentioned in Chapter 1, the definition of exclusive breastfeeding in this paper included up to three 'lapses', or full days of either formula-feeding, or oral rehydration solution, although it did exclude porridge or other solid foods, even if given only once. Nevertheless, even within this very flexible definition, Coovadia and colleagues found that, compared to 'exclusively breastfed' infants, those who had also received formula were twice as likely, and those who received solid foods were 11 times as likely, to become infected through breastmilk.

Compromised infant gut integrity due to mixed feeding

The mechanisms for why exclusive breastfeeding is protective had been well described in a paper published by Melanie Smith and

Louise Kuhn in 2000[17] and by others a decade later.[18,19] They gave the opinion that:

- Supplements given too early interfered with the baby's gut health, even in the first week of life.[20]
- Babies who were infected by three months showed increased gut permeability (leakiness),[21] due to having received early foods, liquids or the use of antibiotics.[22-24]
- Disturbances of the normal gut bacteria were caused by exposure to dietary antigens[21] or inflammation resulting from infections.[25]
- Small sites of trauma and inflammation of the infant's intestinal mucosa[25-27] allowed contact of HIV with the infant's blood supply and immune cells.

The following diagram shows how other foods and liquids can damage the immature baby's gut and why exclusive breastfeeding is protective.

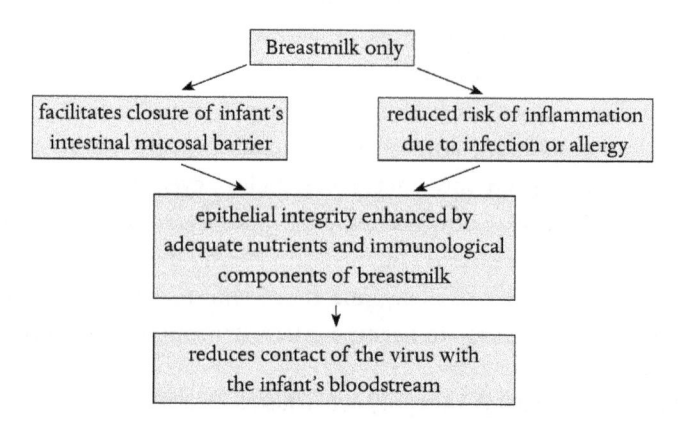

Infant's reduced susceptibility
to HIV with exclusive breastfeeding

Breastmilk only

→ facilitates closure of infant's intestinal mucosal barrier

→ reduced risk of inflammation due to infection or allergy

→ epithelial integrity enhanced by adequate nutrients and immunological components of breastmilk

↓

reduces contact of the virus with the infant's bloodstream

Mixed feeding and/or ineffective breastfeeding may alter the quantity and quality of breastmilk

Mixed feeding can be either a cause or a consequence of a baby not breastfeeding effectively. When the breasts are not well drained, the milk itself may be affected. The milk cells can become permeable, i.e. the 'tight junctions' between breastmilk cells can become disrupted any time that more milk is being made than is being drained from the breast, and before breastmilk production down-regulates. When this happens, milk components can pass into the bloodstream, and lactose, the milk sugar, can actually be measured in the mother's urine.[27] Blood products (including viral particles) can pass into the milk.[28] There is always a time-lag of about four days before the breasts respond to either reduce production (if they're overfull) or increase production (due to being extremely well drained). Over-fullness thus poses a likely risk for elevated HIV viral levels and an increased risk of postnatal transmission of HIV.

Over-fullness may happen as a consequence of:

- A newborn too sleepy to breastfeed effectively, or at all
- Over-production of breastmilk in the first few days after birth
- Feeding the baby other foods or drinks
- A change in the baby's normal feeding pattern, e.g. a missed breastfeed or sleeping longer than usual
- Milk stasis due to a blocked duct or inflammation due to mastitis[26]
- Mother-baby separation
- Fast weaning[29]

The following diagram shows how the combined effect of mixed breastfeeding on the infant gut (infant susceptibility) and on the mother's milk production (maternal infectivity) both exacerbate the risk of mother-to-child transmission of HIV transmission through breastfeeding.

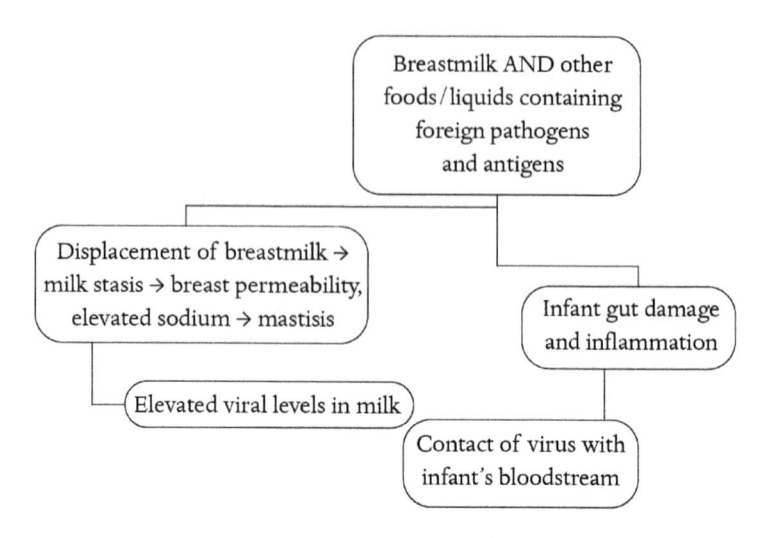

```
                    ┌─────────────────────┐
                    │ Breastmilk AND other│
                    │foods/liquids containing│
                    │  foreign pathogens   │
                    │    and antigens     │
                    └─────────────────────┘
┌──────────────────────────┐      │
│Displacement of breastmilk →│     │
│milk stasis → breast permeability,│     ┌──────────────────┐
│ elevated sodium → mastisis│      │ Infant gut damage │
└──────────────────────────┘      │  and inflammation │
        │                         └──────────────────┘
    ┌────────────────────────┐
    │Elevated viral levels in milk│
    └────────────────────────┘
           ┌──────────────────────┐
           │ Contact of virus with │
           │  infant's bloodstream │
           └──────────────────────┘
```

Morrison P, slide from presentation on How to support First World HIV+ mothers who want to berastfeed. La Leche League of Basque Country, Fourth International Breastfeeding Symposium 'Breastfeeding in Special Circumstances', 15-16 November 2010, Bilbao, Spain.

Which extra foods and liquids are most risky?

In the Coovadia study described earlier in this chapter,[16] infants who were breastfed but also received home-prepared cereal or commercial infant porridges any time after birth were nearly 11 times more likely to acquire HIV infection than exclusively breastfed children. Those who were fed both breastmilk and formula milk at 14 weeks of age had twice the risk. In a Zambian study, when babies were not exclusively breastfed, non-human milk was the most commonly given item other than breastmilk[30] and they rarely received other foods. These babies had a more than three-fold increased risk of early postnatal HIV transmission.

It's thought that proteins found in solid foods cause greater damage to a baby's gastrointestinal lining than the modified cows' milk proteins found in formula. But any kind of damage eases viral entry between cells or alters gut receptors, thereby increasing the likelihood of infection.[16,17]

What can be concluded?
It's crucial to acknowledge:

- the value of exclusive breastfeeding from 0–6 months to protect HIV-exposed babies
- the ability of mothers to exclusively breastfeed; exclusive breastfeeding is not hard when you know how the breasts make milk and how to manage your own lactation.

Mothers appreciate learning how to avoid scenarios that may pose an increased risk of HIV transmission during breastfeeding, so that they are able to manage their own breastmilk supply to make more, or less, as needed. Strategies to accomplish this are set out in Chapter 7. Mixed feeding, while commonly practised, need no longer be used as evidence for the inevitability of transmission of HIV through breastfeeding, since the physiological reasons for it are almost entirely preventable.

Mothers living with HIV need to think about when they will wean
While exclusive breastfeeding is important, it's also an idea to anticipate how your baby will be fed after the first six months come to an end. Will you want to continue breastfeeding after your baby begins taking other foods and liquids at six months, as recommended by WHO? Or will you want to wean completely from the breast? (See chapters 3 and 9.)

Make bottle-feeding familiar if mother-led weaning will be likely (at six months or later)
Babies and toddlers have strong sucking needs which may last for years. Stopping breastfeeding will be easier if your baby is already familiar with bottle-feeding (as mentioned in Chapter 3):

- offer your own milk in a bottle every so often to teach your baby the different skill of bottle-feeding (see Chapter 10 for information on expressing and storing breastmilk)

- be patient as he learns
- some texts suggest that someone else be the one to bottle-feed a breastfed baby, in order that he doesn't become confused and start to prefer the bottle, but you, as the mother, and the person who knows him best, may be the best person to teach him
- for as long as you want to keep on breastfeeding, don't offer the bottle too often or for too long; make bottle-feeds as short as possible so that the baby doesn't get too used to them nor start to prefer the bottle to the breast
- once your baby learns how to bottle-feed, offer a bottle of your own milk every so often to keep up his skills.

SECTION II

HOW BREASTFEEDING WORKS

6. BEGINNING BREASTFEEDING, POSITIONING AND ATTACHMENT, LATCHING TECHNIQUES

Learning to breastfeed

Breastfeeding is not instinctive; it's a learned skill. If you've grown up in a breastfeeding culture where you've always seen family members breastfeeding their babies then you will have learned what to do. In Westernised societies many mothers wistfully observe that breastfeeding an older baby looks so easy, but they may not have had the opportunity to see a newborn at the breast. In the learning period, and as you recover from the birth, you need to be kind to yourself. For the first few weeks you and your baby will need lots of time to perfect your skills, and ideally new mothers should have very few other responsibilities. Getting breastfeeding off to a good start is a very worthwhile investment.

The techniques and protocols for breast and nipple care set out in this book should not be construed as medical advice. They may or may not have exact journal references to support them. In many cases, they are strategies I've honed over many years working with over 3,000 mother-baby pairs, adapted from protocols set out in the lactation literature, learned from other skilled practitioners or taught to me by observing the inventive ways that mothers themselves feed their babies.

Each breastfeeding dyad is individual and unique, with the added dimension that two separate anatomies are involved – the mother's breast and the baby's mouth. No two are alike. If a recommendation doesn't seem to work for your special breast/nipple shape or your baby's mouth, it's okay to try something else. The following suggestions are not rules. They are offered in order of difficulty, the easiest first, e.g. different ways to hold the baby, or to offer the breast, so that the baby can latch, and so that breastfeeding feels comfortable. Feel free to pick what seems to suit you, and if it doesn't work for you and your baby, try another one.

An investment of your time

The early months of breastfeeding are often called the 'fourth trimester' of pregnancy. Human newborns are among the most immature babies of any mammal species. Once a baby has learned to breathe, his second task is to learn to breastfeed – both are life-skills. With patience and persistence, you will be able to

- teach your baby *how* to latch and suckle
- recognise whether he is breastfeeding competently, and
- have some strategies to put in place if he needs a little more help.

In societies where breastfeeding is crucial to child survival, mothers are very patient and persistent about teaching their babies how to latch, and perfect their sucking skills, so that they can obtain enough milk to survive and thrive. In the context of HIV you will not be able to safely top-up with formula supplements because this would mean mixed feeding (which is not recommended, as explained in Chapter 5), so taking the time to bring in a good milk supply is very important. Once you and your baby know what to do, breastfeeding becomes your best mothering tool.

Does your birth experience impact breastfeeding?

A lot is written about how the events surrounding labour and birth affect breastfeeding. How long was the labour, how was the baby delivered, what kind of pain relief did the mother receive? Did she receive intravenous fluids? Will these drugs and fluids sabotage a mother's ability to get off to a good start with breastfeeding and, especially in the context of HIV, will they affect a mother's ability to succeed in breastfeeding exclusively for the first half-year of life?

In areas where breastfeeding rates are low, such as in Europe and America, early events surrounding the birth are frequently given as reasons why breastfeeding is difficult, and why mothers give up breastfeeding before they want to.[1]

Some experts suggest that drugs given during labour (epidural anaesthesia, intravenous fluids, or the pain-killer pethidine) can pose specific difficulties:[2]

- impair a baby's ability to suck
- disturb the mother's milk-ejection reflex
- exacerbate newborn weight loss in the first few days of life by pumping the baby full of extra fluids during labour, which he loses in the first 24 hours

But do these medications always pose insurmountable challenges to breastfeeding? Probably not. It's important to stress that if you need pain relief or certain procedures during your labour, you should have them. In countries where breastfeeding is universally practised, events during labour or the type of birth don't prevent breastfeeding. Breastfeeding begins when labour and delivery are over. Doctors, nursing staff and mothers put in place strategies and protocols to work around and through any of these events so that breastfeeding can be initiated with the least delay in spite of them.

Breastfeeding in the first hour after birth

It's a great help if you and your baby can enjoy skin-to-skin contact as soon as possible after birth. Ask if your baby can be placed on your abdomen or chest between your breasts. During the first hour or two a newborn is usually in a heightened alert state and his sucking instinct is particularly strong, so taking advantage of this window of opportunity to offer the breast for the first time is ideal. Within 20 minutes or so of birth, your baby may start to crawl upwards and bob around to find your nipple and attach to the breast. This self-attachment journey has been named the 'breast crawl'.[3] If you are not able to see what your baby is doing if you're on your back you can either allow your baby to complete the breast crawl and attach by himself, or you can ask your midwives or your partner to help him find the breast.

If there's a delay in the first breastfeed

While there is so much written and said about the importance of the magic hour after birth, there may be constraints which delay or prevent it. Nursing staff may be required to wipe or clean vernix and fluids from an HIV-exposed baby. If something happens to prevent you offering the breast immediately, it may be disappointing, but just go with the hospital protocol and begin breastfeeding as soon as you can. If your baby has to be taken away to another room for washing, ask if you or the baby's father are able to stay with him. Needless to say, he should not be allowed to become distressed or chilled, and should not be fed any other milks or liquids during his time away from you. This is where a breastfeeding plan, previously signed off by your doctors, can back up your wishes. If something delays the first breastfeed, then you simply begin breastfeeding as soon as you can.

Basic rules

Breastfeeding is like a dance: once you and your baby know the steps it's easy. There are only a few basic moves to get started:

1. Hold the baby tummy to tummy with you so that he can reach the breast
2. His ear, shoulder and hip should be in a straight line, so he is not twisted
3. Tickle his lips very lightly with your nipple
4. Wait for him to open his mouth wide in a yawn
5. Quickly bring him on to your breast
6. Breastfeed him for as long as he wants and as often as he wants.

General tips

When your newborn baby is very tiny, it helps if you can make positioning as easy as possible for him and as comfortable as possible for you. There is no hard and fast rule for how to hold him for breastfeeding. As long as he can reach the breast, you can breastfeed in any position that you find comfortable. The baby's tummy should be as close to your body as possible, and he should be well supported so that he can use his energy to breastfeed, rather than to stabilise himself. He should not have to turn his head to breastfeed (try and swallow with your chin pointed towards your shoulder and you will see why this is important…)

As your baby grows and as you both become more experienced, you will find that you can breastfeed anywhere, any time, without giving it a thought. Older babies and toddlers help themselves, and often breastfeed standing up, upside down, or in other funny or annoying positions (depending on your point of view).

Working with your baby's reflexes

Babies have a few innate reflexes and survival mechanisms and it can save a lot of frustration if you know how to work along with them as you position and latch your baby to your breast:

- Babies will turn their heads towards any stimulus on the face. So if your fingers, or even a blanket or a piece of clothing touches his cheeks or face, he will turn towards it, even frustratingly turning *away* from the breast and towards a blanket or a finger touching his cheek. The more you attempt to push him towards the breast, the stronger he will push away from it. Make sure nothing is touching his cheeks!
- Babies cannot swallow if their heads are turned. Hold your baby tummy to tummy with you, with his ear, shoulder and hip in a straight line, *not* turning his head.
- Babies become frantic and arch *away* from the breast if the backs of their heads are held or pushed (as you might think of doing to enable him to reach your breast). He needs his back and shoulders to be supported, and you can bring him close to you, or lift him higher or lower by supporting his *neck with your fingers behind and below his ears*. Do not push on the back of his head!
- A very hungry baby will clench his fists or grab anything he can to bring it to his mouth and this can make latching difficult

because his arms will be held tight to his chest. You need his chest to be clear and as close to your body as possible. You can tuck his underneath arm around you and then allow his top arm to rest on your breast. If you just can't manage this you can swaddle him with his arms by his sides. Generally speaking, though, it's better for him to be able to feel your breast so that he can make the little patting and squeezing movements that baby mammals use to help the mother's milk flow faster.
- A crying baby is very hard to latch. While his mouth is open – which you would think would make offering the breast easier – his tongue will be elevated towards his top gum, so that he cannot take the nipple into his mouth. It's helpful to offer the breast before he becomes too hungry or frustrated (don't change the nappy first, change it afterwards... and have everything ready to breastfeed, bra undone, and everything you need available, so he doesn't have to wait).
- You can calm a crying baby by holding him upright against your shoulder and patting or rocking him until he calms down, then *quickly* put him in position and offer the breast again.
- Babies need to feel something along the palate (roof of the mouth), not on the back of the tongue (which will make him gag) to know that there is a nipple there to suck.[4]
- Babies may arch backwards if there is any pressure on their feet, so whatever position you use, make sure that you don't have any surfaces that he can push against. Try bending him at the hips and curling his body around you, or have his legs resting up along the back of the chair, avoiding pressure on his feet.
- Babies also stiffen and arch backwards and scream if they are hungry or angry and frustrated. The breast is your best mothering tool. Any time you don't know what is wrong with the baby, offer the breast again.
- Babies love to use the breast for comfort and to go to sleep with. A baby may take 20 minutes to fall into a deep sleep and become frustrated if you take him off the breast too soon, or if you wake him up unnecessarily (e.g. to burp him when he

is 'milk-drunk' and sleepy). It's always appropriate to offer the breast again. And again…

Your comfort

Your newborn may only weigh 3kg at birth, but after ten minutes of holding him up to your breast, it starts to feel like a lot more. Little babies may also take quite a long time to feed, so it's a good idea to use pillows to support the baby, or your arm, under your knees, behind your back or wherever feels most comfortable. Ordinary soft, squishy cushions or bed pillows may work better than commercially manufactured nursing pillows which are often very firm. All that matters is that your baby can breastfeed easily, and that you should be so comfortable that, once he is latched nicely, you can completely relax all your muscles and be sure that he won't slip.

Positioning

You can hold your baby in any one of several ways. Several organisations have written about, or produced useful videos showing different breastfeeding positions.[5-7]

Cradle hold *

In this position you cradle your baby in your arms. This is probably the most popular breastfeeding position. It is sometimes called the 'Madonna hold' because it is so often shown in old religious paintings. It's helpful to use a pillow under your arm or on your lap to support the baby. In the cradle hold:

---

* The images in this chapter, except where indicated, are from WHO 2009, *Infant and young child feeding: model chapter for textbooks for medical students and allied health professionals*. ISBN 978924159749

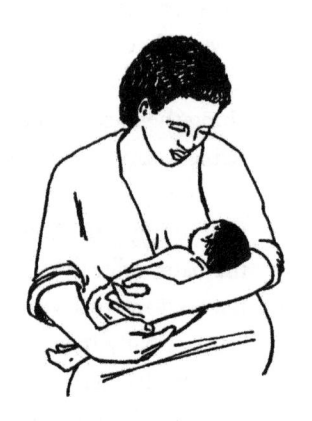

- you are sitting up, or sitting cross-legged
- the baby is held in the crook of your arm, tummy to tummy with you
- you lean forward a little to latch the baby (the angle of dangle of your breast makes it more pointy and graspable and this makes latching easier)
- offer the breast of the same side, e.g. *left* breast, *left* arm)
- support the breast with the opposite (*right*) hand
- once the baby is latched and sucking happily, then lean back a little for your own comfort, but continue to support the breast well.

Cross-cradle hold

This is a very good position to use if you need to take extra care (e.g. the baby is tricky to latch, or your nipples are becoming tender) because you have excellent control over exactly where your baby's mouth latches as he takes the breast:

- hold the baby tummy to tummy with you
- if holding the baby on your *left*, offer the *left* breast with your *left* hand
- hold the baby with the opposite hand, e.g. *left* breast, *right* hand
- support the baby's upper back and neck with your palm and support his neck with your thumb and forefinger spread *below* and *behind* his ears

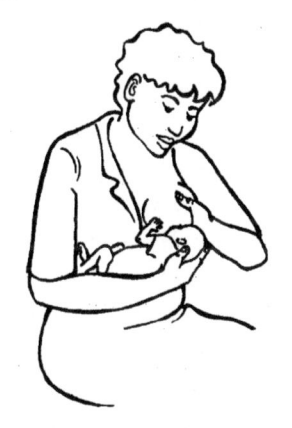

WHO 1993, Breastfeeding Counselling: a Training Course, Participants Manual.

- once the baby is latched comfortably and sucking well, you can either
    > stay in that position, with a pillow under your *left* elbow so that you can lean into it comfortably, or
    > carefully change over to the *cradle hold*; slowly and gently let go of the breast with your *left* hand, place your left arm

around your baby (as in the cradle hold), then remove your *right* hand from the baby's back and neck and slip it under your breast for support. When changing hands like this you need to move carefully and slowly to avoid inadvertently unlatching him and having to start all over again.

Rugby hold or football hold
In this position you hold the baby as if you are carrying a rugby ball, or an American football. It's a useful position if you need to see what you're doing, and need more control. It can also be a very comfortable position for simultaneously breastfeeding twins, or for breastfeeding your single baby while you play with your older toddler sitting beside you on the other side:

- have the baby beside you, held close to your body with the arm and hand of the same side (e.g. *right* breast, *right* arm)
- use pillows beside you and across your body to lift the baby so that his mouth is in line with your nipple
- have his head facing forward and his feet tucked behind under your arm
- support his upper back with the palm of your hand
- support his neck with your thumb and index finger spread below and behind his ears, don't touch his face or the back of his head
- ensure that the baby's feet are not pushing against the back of the chair
- lean forward a little for latching
- support your *right* breast with your *left* hand

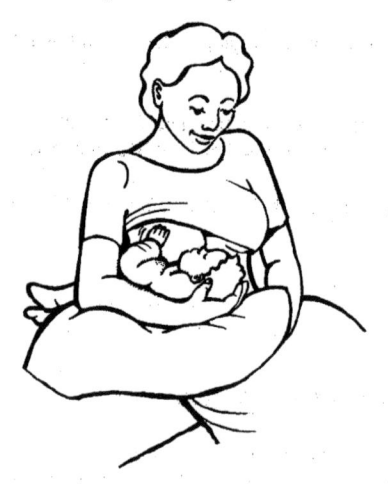

WHO 1993, Breastfeeding Counselling: a Training Course, Participants Manual.

- once latched, you can lean back slowly, tuck the pillows comfortably and perhaps support your raised foot on a footstool but continue to support the breast.

Koala hold
This can be a useful hold if you think your baby may be spitting up a lot, or if he has a blocked nose or difficulty breathing while breastfeeding:

- if offering the *left* breast hold your baby upright, straddling your *left* thigh and facing you
- support his back and neck with your *left* hand
- ensure the baby's spine is straight and not slumped
- offer the breast with your *right* hand
- support your arms with pillows for comfort so you can relax, and remember to drop your shoulders.

Laid-back breastfeeding
This is sometimes called 'biological nurturing'.[8] For laid-back breastfeeding:

- half recline on a comfortable chair/sofa/bed, with enough pillows so that your back and arm are well supported
- hold the baby tummy to tummy with you, positioned diagonally across your body, so he can reach the nipple
- allow the baby to self-attach
- gravity keeps the baby in position.

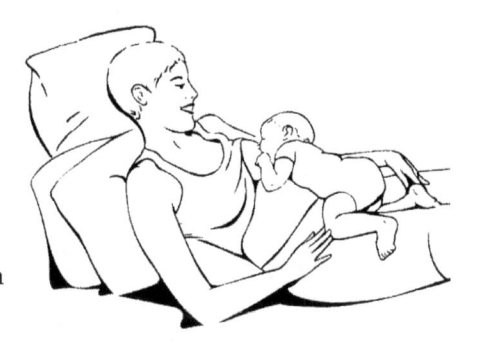

Image: LLLUSA lllusa.org/lie-back-and-relax-a-look-at-laid-back-breastfeeding

This position is highly promoted in the lactation community since it's believed to facilitate breastfeeding by working with normal mammal reflexes.[9] However, while many mammal mothers feed their babies lying down, primates usually sit up, as do unsophisticated human mothers in resource-poor settings who don't own stuffed furniture or pillows on which to recline. My observation is that this position may be less helpful while you're learning to breastfeed because the breast tends to flatten and spread when the mother lies back, *and* she can't see where the baby's mouth is placed. Laid back breastfeeding may be more comfortable and easier when the baby grows older.

Side-lying
This position can also be a little tricky to master for a new mother, but it's a very useful position, because you can snooze at the same time.

- lie down on your side, with your head on one or two pillows or resting on your raised arm
- have a pillow down your back to lean into slightly, and another between your knees for balance
- position your baby beside you, with his nose level with your nipple and his chest and abdomen close to your body; ear, shoulder and hip in a straight line
- gently guide him on to the breast so that once latched his head is tipped back a little

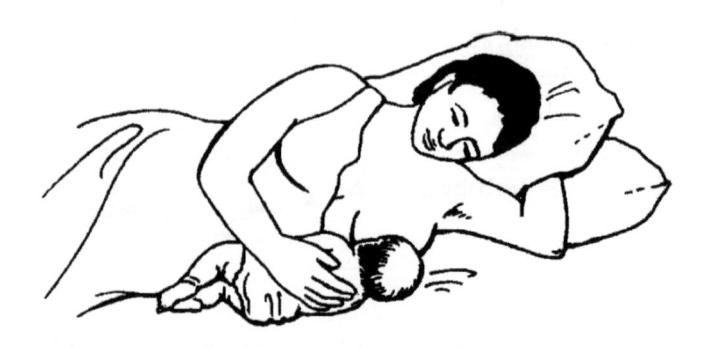

- support your baby's upper back and neck with the palm of your hand or a rolled up towel so he doesn't roll on to his back
- change sides by holding the baby to your chest and rolling over taking him with you, then re-latch on to the other breast
- mothers with very large breasts may be able to offer the upper breast without changing their own position

Attachment (latching your baby)

The way the baby latches to the breast profoundly affects how much milk he can obtain, as well as the mother's comfort and nipple health. When you're aiming for exclusive breastfeeding for a full six months, where and how the baby suckles is really important. Once he's latched, his chin should be dug well in to the breast below the areola, and his nose should be just touching above.

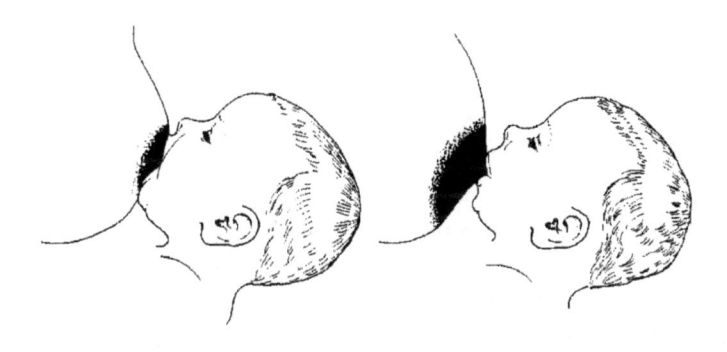

Good attachment (left)   Poor attachment (right)

Stimulating your baby to open his mouth

If a baby is ready to feed, he will open his mouth wide like a yawn (a gape) if anything brushes his lips. To take the breast into his mouth, he needs to have a wide open mouth and his tongue needs to be down. You can encourage him to drop his tongue by brushing his *lower* lip with your nipple. If you mash your nipple against his lips he may clamp his mouth firmly shut. You need to be subtle – just lightly tickle his lower lip, wait a millisecond for him to open, and then quickly bring him on to the breast. Babies have slightly receding chins so he should attach to the breast with what is called an *asymmetric latch* – with more of the underside of the areola in his mouth than the top.

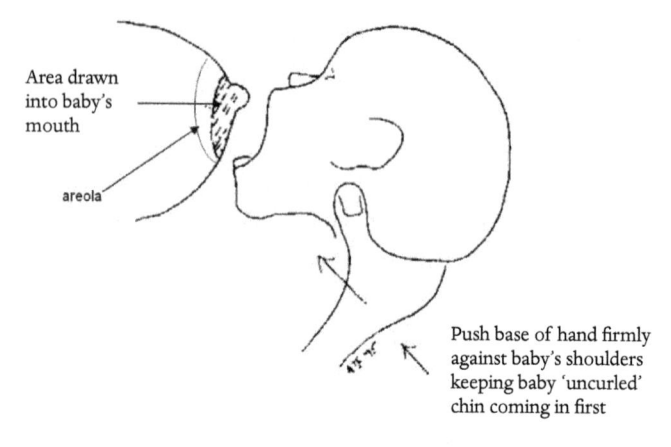

Area drawn into baby's mouth

areola

Push base of hand firmly against baby's shoulders keeping baby 'uncurled' chin coming in first

Image: courtesy Dr Jack Newman, from Ann Barnes, and latching info at ibconline.ca/information-sheets/latching-and-feeding

How to support your breast

Many mothers breastfeed their babies, especially if they are older, without providing any support for the breast at all. If the baby can latch and if, after latching, breastfeeding is comfortable for you, then breast support is certainly not essential. However, while you and your baby are learning, it seems to be easier to give the baby as much help as possible. At first, supporting the heavy breast throughout the feed takes the weight off his lower jaw and helps him to stay attached, as well as avoiding nipple pain and damage for the mother.

The C-hold

Most breastfeeding specialists recommend supporting the breast in a 'C' hold:

- cup your breast with your fingers under the areola (the dark tissue around the nipple), and your thumb on top, leaving room

for the baby's mouth to cover the nipple and some of the areola
- stimulate the baby to open his mouth by tickling his lips very gently with the tip of your nipple (if you do this too hard he may clamp his gums shut…)
- then *wait* for him to gape (i.e. open his mouth as wide as a yawn)
- Then, with a rapid movement of the arm or hand holding the baby, quickly bring his mouth over your nipple (i.e. move the baby, not the breast) and wait for a little tug on your nipple which tells you he has latched
- the baby needs to take a nice big mouthful of breast tissue into his mouth as he latches, i.e. the whole nipple and some of the areola.

Support your breast throughout the feed

- once latched, the baby's chin should be dug well into the breast below the areola, and the nose should be just touching the breast on top.[10] Babies have flattened little noses so that they are able to breathe as long as the nostrils are not completely blocked by breast tissue. If in doubt, pull the baby's bottom in a little closer to your body; this will tip his nose out a little more.
- don't put a finger on top of the breast to make an airway – this blocks some of the milk producing ducts, stretches the areolar tissue and brings the nipple forward in his mouth. A baby with a weak suck will let go. A baby with a strong suck will hang on and this can cause stretching, leading to sore nipples, something you want to avoid.
- be sure to *support* the heavy breast well from underneath *throughout the feed*. When the baby is little, this takes the weight of the heavy breast off his lower jaw, and flattens the underside of the breast, enabling him to take and maintain a deeper latch, and to milk the breast more effectively. Imagine that you are 'pouring' the breast into the baby's mouth, from the back.
- You can assess whether the baby is placed well on the breast by looking at the breast tissue near the areola. If it's moving in and out with each suck, then without unlatching the baby, you need

to adjust something – usually by moving the baby towards the stretching, or by moving the breast slightly towards the baby's mouth.
- As the feed progresses you may find that the baby slips (he's heavy!) and begins to 'drag' on the breast and this also can cause stretching (as described above). Support the breast well and make an adjustment so that this no longer happens.

Experimenting with different latching techniques

If your baby is struggling to latch, or if you are becoming sore, there are several different latching techniques that can help your baby, or make latching more comfortable for you. You can add them to your toolbox of breastfeeding skills. Babies learn incredibly quickly, and while your little one might need help on day one after birth, he will probably behave like an old pro in a week, so that you almost certainly won't need to use these somewhat cumbersome techniques forever. Within just a few days, you and your baby will find your own best way together and you will not always need to be so careful.

Pointing the nipple upwards

This is a tip that can prove very useful for a baby who seems to be difficult to latch because it is stimulation to the roof of the baby's mouth which causes him to 'latch':

- cup your breast in the 'C' hold as above, all four fingers underneath, thumb on top
- dig your thumb in a little above the areola so that the nipple points upwards and so that the underside of the areola seems to enter his mouth first
- draw him on to the breast quickly before he becomes frustrated
- once he is latched, slowly release the pressure on your thumb so that he can draw the nipple far back into his mouth where it won't become damaged
- Continue to support the breast from underneath as if you are 'pouring' the breast into the baby's mouth.

Scissors hold

This is a way of holding the breast commonly used by mothers living in Third World countries where breastfeeding is the cultural norm. It's not favoured by specialists living in the First World who prefer the 'C' hold, but it can firm up the breast tissue, and make the nipple more protuberant. This can make latching easier for babies who might (temporarily) need to feel something firmer before they know what to do. For scissors:

- cup the breast with the third, fourth and fifth fingers under the areola
- leave the index finger on top above
- firm the breast tissue by pulling slightly back towards the ribs; pulling back like this makes the nipple stick out a little more
- the nipple can be directed up towards the baby's palate by slightly digging the index finger into the breast tissue
- once the baby is latched, slowly let go the backward pressure, but continue to support the breast from underneath.

The nipple sandwich

This useful technique, often used with the cross-cradle position, assists with latching by firming the areolar tissue to make the nipple more graspable, effectively presenting the breast to the baby as if it is a sandwich or hamburger. By flattening the rounded underneath of the breast the baby's lower jaw can take more of the underneath in, which gives a deeper latch:

- support the breast with a flat index finger underneath and slightly behind the areola (leaving room for the baby's chin) *in line with his smile*
- stimulate him to gape wide by tickling his lips very softly with the tip of the nipple
- bring him on to the firmed breast tissue by ensuring he comes on chin first

- 'plant' the underside of the areola on to the baby's tongue and keep the breast well supported throughout the breastfeed.

The flipple

This technique flips the nipple into the baby's mouth. Also used with the cross-cradle position, it's an exaggerated way of pointing the nipple up to provide good stimulation to the baby's palate. It's a useful position to use if the baby is having difficulty finding the breast or to achieve a deeper latch to resolve sore nipples:

- use the sandwich hold to support the breast, with your underside fingers in line with the baby's smile
- slightly dig the thumb into the breast tissue on top, which will tilt the nipple up
- tickle the baby's lips to stimulate the gape *with the underside of the areola*
- wait till he gapes wide, then plant the underside of the areola on the baby's tongue
- as you latch him, release the pressure of your thumb, allowing the nipple to flip into the baby's mouth, along the palate, as shown in the IABLE[11] and Global Health Media videos.[12]

The tea-cup hold

If a baby is finding it really hard to latch, or if your nipples are a little flat, the tea-cup hold for the nipple and areola allows you to place the nipple up into his palate so that he can't fail to feel it. This is a very delicate technique, and you'll need some skill to pull it off, but once your baby knows what to do, you probably won't need to latch in this way more than once or twice – babies learn very quickly and he may learn in only one or two helping sessions how to draw your nipple up into his palate all by himself. It's easier if you have very elastic areolar tissue. It's very difficult if your breasts are too full – you will have to express some milk first to soften the breast and especially the areola.

- position the baby in a cross-cradle hold
- support the breast underneath with your middle, fourth and fifth finger
- with your index finger and thumb, take a pinch of the areolar tissue *beside* the nipple, using the skin of the areola as a sort of nipple handle
- stimulate the baby's gape by lightly brushing his lower lip with your nipple and wait until he opens his mouth wide like a yawn, with his tongue down
- using the handle you've created, stretch the nipple as far back into his mouth as you can, and put the tip of the nipple *up so that it touches the baby's palate* and he can feel that it's there
- once he can feel the stimulus, the baby will latch on to the nipple
- as the baby takes the first suck, and tugs on your nipple, quickly release your tea-cup hold on the areola, and move your fingers out of the baby's mouth *but keep supporting your breast underneath with your middle, fourth and fifth finger*
- try not to move anything else until you can see that your baby is sucking and swallowing competently.

Babies who forget how to latch

When babies who have been latching and breastfeeding for several days suddenly seem to forget what to do, it can be very disconcerting. There are two likely causes:

- The breasts may have become very engorged, flattening the nipple and areola. If this happens, the engorgement needs to be dealt with very promptly by pumping enough milk to soften the breast and areola, so that you can try latching again. In the meantime the baby can receive expressed breastmilk (see Chapter 10) until he can resume breastfeeding.
- The mother may have had the painkiller pethidine quite close to delivery. This drug can negatively affect the baby's sucking skills for about 10 days. An antidote called naloxone is sometimes given to the baby to offset the effects of the pethidine, so the

baby seems to latch easily and breastfeeding seems to go well, but the effects of naloxone wear off after three days and it seems as if suddenly the baby 'unlearns' how to suck. The solution is to pump and feed him expressed breastmilk for a week or so, keep trying him at the breast and just wait until the pethidine wears off and he reacquires his sucking skills.

Suck training

If the baby continually seems to be confused about taking the breast, you can try a little suck training. Offer him a clean finger to suck, pad side up towards his palate, and let him suck for a minute or two until he is calm and ready to try latching again. Don't push down on his tongue because that will make him gag. Then you can get comfortable, take a deep breath, withdraw your finger and offer the breast again straight away before he becomes upset. Repeat as necessary. If your partner is helping, have him offer his pinky finger while you get comfortable. Sometimes it takes several people to latch one upset baby.

Nipple confusion

Sometimes babies who have experienced latching difficulties are believed to experience 'nipple confusion' due to having been bottle-fed before they have learned to breastfeed. However, remember that mothers who want to breastfeed usually only offer the baby a bottle as a last resort and only after he has already failed to latch to the breast. Thus it may be that nipple confusion is a consequence, not a cause, of a breastfeeding difficulty.

Bottles can also sometimes be used as a form of suck training for a baby who has not yet learned what to do. Once a difficult-to-latch baby has been bottle-fed breastmilk in sufficient quantities to satisfy his growing appetite so that he becomes calm and relaxed, it may be surprisingly easy to simply offer the breast and see what happens. Most babies go on to the breast like a dream.

To make the change from bottle to breast:
- read the positioning and latching recommendations above. Choose the position that seems most likely to work for you and your baby
- have a bottle of expressed breastmilk handy in case the baby becomes upset
- offer the breast by gently tickling his lips, waiting for him to gape and bringing him on to the breast quickly (as described above) and ensuring that his palate is stimulated, i.e. your nipple is pointing *up*.
- reward the baby with big smiles for even one or two sucks, don't hurry him, wait for him to carry on
- most babies will start sucking and simply continue
- if he can't seem to latch, try a couple of times, but stop when he shows he is becoming frustrated, offer the bottle and try again another time
- if you experience further difficulty, call an IBCLC for a face-to-face consult so that you can receive one-to-one recommendations tailored especially to your breast/nipple shape and the baby's oral anatomy.

Persistent latching difficulty

Most babies learn how to breastfeed very quickly, the first time they are offered the breast. Some babies, though, seem to need more opportunities for learning, and may take 2–3 days to learn what to do. Perhaps the birth was difficult and the baby needs time to recover. The mother's breast and nipple shape and size make a difference; short nipples may be less graspable, or the nipples may even be flat or inverted. The baby's oral anatomy may be challenging. Some babies have a prominent upper gum ridge or a high palate which makes latching more difficult. Sometimes it's a combination of several things, which a colleague describes as the 'the oro-boobular fit'![13] The possibility of latching difficulties due to a baby having a tongue-tie has gained currency in recent years. Please see Chapter 13 for more information about the importance of *not* performing a frenotomy (tongue-tie release) on an HIV-exposed baby.

As described above, in order to latch, the baby needs to feel the nipple *up* along his *palate*. If he can't feel stimulation to the roof of his mouth, he doesn't know that the breast is there.[4] Oddly enough, when he's searching for the nipple it can look as if he's refusing the breast, opening his mouth and shaking his head from side to side, like a dog worrying a bone. This behaviour can be confusing and frustrating to the mother. Babies stiffen and arch when they're frustrated and if a baby is becoming upset because he can't find the nipple, he will cry and arch backwards *away* from the breast. Mothers sometimes interpret this to mean that the baby is saying 'no', or rejecting them. Not so! Review the suggestions above. Once he can feel something stimulating the roof of his mouth, he will go on to the breast, close his mouth around it, stop flailing around, and then take an exploratory suck, and then another and then start sucking rhythmically, and you have success!

Getting more help

If latching continues to be difficult, consider temporary use of a nipple shield (see Chapter 13).

If difficulties persist, start expressing and feeding your colostrum or expressed breastmilk (see Chapter 10) and call your IBCLC for a face-to-face consult for more tailor-made suggestions.

7. LACTATION MANAGEMENT FOR MOTHERS

Understanding breastmilk production

Breastfeeding is a system that is meant to work. During late pregnancy and for the first 2–3 days after birth, the breasts produce a protein-rich early milk called colostrum. The quantity of colostrum secreted in the first 24 hours is about six teaspoonfuls. The small quantity is a huge advantage for the inexperienced baby. He is able to learn how to simultaneously suck, swallow and breathe, and perfect these skills, by frequent practice sessions on a breast that is producing only tiny amounts of milk. This scanty but precious liquid gold, high in antibodies, coats the baby's gut to boost his immune system against invasion by bacteria, viruses and fungi.

Within just a few days of birth, 99.9% of mothers will begin to produce the daily 750–900ml of breastmilk that their babies are going to need.[1] In a perfect example of demand-creation, the breasts will continue to make milk, store it, release it and refill, enabling a healthy, growing baby to survive and thrive on mother's milk alone for the first half-year of life. But Nature abhors waste. If the milk is not taken or drained from the breasts, production will slow down and eventually cease, as described in Chapter 5.

Breastmilk synthesis is a dynamic process

Breastmilk production is not static. The quantity varies:

- from woman to woman
- between breasts in the same woman
- from day to day
- between morning and evening
- from hour to hour

Some women have a large breastmilk storage capacity within their breasts and would only need to breastfeed about three times a day for their babies to receive enough milk. Others with a smaller storage capacity might need to breastfeed 20 times in 24 hours to keep their babies well fed. But each mother can maximise her own individual ability to make enough milk for her baby, or for twins, or even for triplets.

Initiation of breastmilk production

An understanding of a few basic principles will enable every mother to breastfeed safely so as to reduce the risk of transmission of HIV to the breastfed baby to virtually zero.

At various times, a mother may want to:

- start breastfeeding
- produce enough milk to exclusively breastfeed for a full six months
- maintain, increase or decrease her breastmilk supply
- stop breastfeeding altogether

Lactogenesis I and II

The easiest method of bringing in a breastmilk supply is to become pregnant and give birth to a baby. Before birth, your uterus creates a safe, protective, warm environment for your baby to grow until he is mature enough to exist independently. The baby is a parasite, channelling what he needs – food, fluids, and even oxygen – from the mother's body, through his placenta and into his own bloodstream. And while this is happening, the placenta, which is foetal (not maternal) tissue, exerts hormonal influences on the mother's breasts, causing the ducts and cells to grow and divide and then to produce milk (to lactate) to feed him after he is born.

One of the first signs of pregnancy is tender breasts and there's a reason for this. Oestrogen and progesterone released by the placenta cause the breast tissue, which began developing during puberty, to proliferate into numerous lobes and ducts ending in little bunches of grape-like milk-producing structures known as alveoli.[2] Thus, if the baby is born any time after the 16th week of pregnancy the breasts are ready to begin producing milk (called Lactogenesis I). In a marvel of forward planning, the baby effectively assures his own continuing food supply a whole 24 weeks before his due date, well before he could even hope to survive outside his mother's body.

In a further clever interplay of hormonal influences, the milk-producing hormone prolactin, necessary for complete growth of the mammary gland, is secreted in high quantities during late pregnancy by the mother's anterior pituitary gland. Progesterone over-rides the action of prolactin, to act as a brake on milk production until needed by the baby after birth. After expulsion of the baby's placenta (also aptly known as the 'afterbirth') it is the sudden withdrawal, or *absence* of progesterone, that lifts the brake and allows milk to be made in increasing quantities. This process is called Lactogenesis II or the milk 'coming in'.

From 36–72 hours after birth, regardless of any action the mother may take, and whether she chooses to breastfeed or not, milk production increases dramatically. The taste changes from salty to sweet as the protein and sodium content of colostrum decreases and the sugar content rises, leading to an increase in the water content and volume. From the third or fourth day the mother will usually gradually become aware that the breasts are starting to feel hot, heavy and increasingly full. Ideally, if a baby is breastfeeding well, this process may be so subtle that she may not be aware of increasing milk production unless she notices that the baby is swallowing more milk.

Lactogenesis II is the pivotal phase for a mother who wants to be successful at breastfeeding. The reason is that during the first and second weeks, there can be something of a mismatch between your milk production and your baby's intake. Once the milk comes in the breasts are initially geared towards producing a lot of milk, probably more than enough for just one baby, as if Nature doesn't know that you didn't have twins. Good breast care during this time will pay dividends in the future.

The volume of milk that you produce increases dramatically at this time. There is the potential to produce more milk than your baby needs, especially from days 4–9 following the birth, as explained further below. His appetite may lag behind, causing you to become too full. In addition, there is always a four-day time-lag with breasts; if you become too full on Monday, your breasts may not slow production in any noticeable way until Friday and, if you do nothing to increase drainage, you can become fuller and fuller. This is one reason why it's important to make sure that the baby is breastfeeding effectively, right from the beginning, and if not, that you know how to provide self-care for your breasts, as described below and in Chapter 12.

Milk transfer to the baby

The purpose of breastfeeding is, of course, to feed the baby. The baby's warm mouth on the mother's breast will usually trigger her posterior pituitary gland to release oxytocin, which acts on small basket-like cells surrounding milk-producing alveoli in the breast, to squeeze milk into the ducts and make it available to the baby. This is called the milk-ejection/let-down reflex. Once this reflex becomes well established, it's almost impossible to disturb, and can be triggered by the sight, sound, smell or even the thought of the baby.

Babies who are learning to breastfeed may latch and then wait a little before starting to suck, as if they're checking things out first. Be patient. That warm little mouth is sending signals to your posterior pituitary gland to facilitate the let-down. Sometimes you can detect that the baby's jaw gives a subtle little tremor, and this tiny stimulation is also enough to cause your milk to start flowing. Thus either partner in the breastfeeding relationship can trigger the milk to flow so that the baby can drink. Babies can appear to doze at the breast if there is no milk flowing. When it does, they will open their eyes and breastfeed with great concentration.

As the baby's jaw drops during suckling (called a jaw excursion) a vacuum is created inside the baby's mouth. The oral vacuum helps milk to flow freely from the breast, which ejects milk whenever oxytocin release pushes milk from the ducts down towards the nipple. An ineffective seal, due to a cleft palate or other oral issues, or to a heavy breast dragging on the baby's lower jaw, will make for difficulty feeding.

You can monitor milk transfer from your breast to your baby by watching his jaw movements and swallowing:

- When only a little milk is being transferred your newborn will take short, quick sucks, e.g. suck-suck-suck, suck-suck-suck. Then rest and begin again.
- Most babies will take a few quick sucks, to trigger a let-down; suck-suck-suck, and then wait, and then a few more shallow (not fully jaw-dropping) sucks, and another wait, and then they start drinking as the milk flows freely. Some babies pull away if milk does not instantly appear, but will return eagerly to try again, until the milk does start to flow.
- When your milk is flowing, the rhythm of the baby's suckling changes, becoming much slower. The baby's jaw drops further and opens wide before each long, slow swallow, and there is tiny pause at the peak of each jaw excursion.
    > You can see swallowing happening, e.g. chomp – open – pause – swallow, chomp – open – pause – swallow, chomp – open – pause – swallow...
    > Or you can hear swallowing, which usually sounds like a soft C, C, C...
    > Dr Jack Newman, a very experienced Canadian breastfeeding expert and paediatrician, has a website where he shares videos of latching, sucking and swallowing.
- Sucking bursts usually consist of up to 10 swallows followed by a rest while the baby stays attached, then the baby will trigger the mother's breast to let down more milk, and there will be another sucking burst and then another small rest. As the feed on each breast progresses, there will likely be fewer swallows in each sucking burst, as the volume and speed of milk transfer slows down.

- Over the first couple of weeks, as your milk production increases, you will notice that the baby swallows more. A very full breast will push milk out faster, sometimes so fast the baby cannot keep up, and comes off spluttering.
- Interestingly, the size of the newborn swallow is said to be on average only 0.6ml, so it may take a while for a newborn baby to feel full. (This varies, so please don't start counting swallows and calculating volumes!)
- Allow your baby to drink as long as he wants and to self-detach when he loses interest in suckling on the first breast, then offer the second breast.
- Longer feed times are good for little babies; being close to the mother's body provides the baby with temperature regulation and reduction of stress, and helps his immune system to function more efficiently. Babies become much faster feeders as they grow – sometimes a full feed takes only 10 minutes or less for older babies.
- Generally speaking, the emptier the breast, the richer the cream content of the milk. Milk fat is important for the normal development of the brain and nervous system, as well as for growth. The baby fed ad lib will regulate his fat intake. Hungrier babies will stay longer at a seemingly 'empty' breast (although the lactating breast is never truly empty, there is always some milk left, so trust your baby to feed as long as he wants).
- When babies are hungry they have high muscle tone, holding their arms close to their bodies and their fists up to their mouths. You can know that your baby is not full by trying to lift his elbow away from his body. Even if he appears to be asleep he will feel tight and resist you. Conversely, when he's full, he will relax; if you try to lift his arm it will be floppy. Allow him to breastfeed as long as he wants.
- Babies have evolved to grow fat fast, as a survival strategy. A solely breastfed baby cannot be overfed.[4]

The suck/swallow pattern of a feed

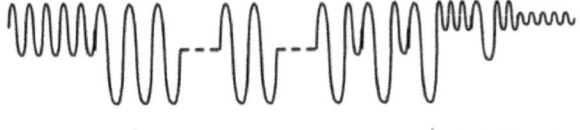

| Beginning of feed - short, rapid sucks | Active feeding - long, slow, rhythmic sucking and swallowing, with pauses | End of feed - 'flutter sucking' with occasional swallows |

Adapted from Minchin MK Breastfeeding Matters: what we need to know about infant feeding. Alma Publications, 4th edition, p.102.

How long is a breastfeed? (feeding duration)

As they are learning to perfect their breastfeeding skills, newborns need to be trusted to know how long to feed. A small baby may want to feed little and often, and it's best if you allow him lots of practice. The longer a small newborn is allowed to suck, the more regulated his behaviour becomes and the calmer he seems. As he becomes more competent, and learns what to do, he may stay on the breast for longer and lengthen the intervals between breastfeeds.

- Young babies will probably need to suck for 20–30 minutes, in order to get enough milk.
- Allow the baby to breastfeed as long as he wants on the first breast.
- Let him have a short rest and then offer the second breast.
- At certain times, the baby may be satisfied with one breast (a snack, or a quick drink).
- At other times, he may want a five-course meal, cluster-feeding several times over a couple of hours, and then sleeping for a couple of hours.
- The water content of the milk is highest when the breast is most full and lowest when the breast is more emptied. Based on a study conducted in 1988,[5] this phenomenon is sometimes interpreted as meaning that the breast makes two different kinds of milk, 'foremilk' and 'hindmilk'. This is an unfortunate

myth; what happens is that the fat content of the milk *gradually* increases as the breast becomes more drained. Allow your baby to 'finish the first breast first', and to feed as long as he wants on either breast.

- Generally speaking, it's best to alternate breasts, but you can also offer the fullest breast first, whichever that is.
- Most mothers observe that one breast is more efficient at making milk than the other, usually in a 60%–40% ratio. Often, but not always, the right breast is slightly larger and makes more milk. Be reassured that this is normal.
- Babies may feed for shorter times in the mornings when milk volume is higher and may want to cluster-feed in the late afternoon or evenings when milk production seems to slow down. Trust him.
- Older babies may drain a breast pretty thoroughly in five minutes, but they may want to go on sucking for much longer because it feels so delicious.

How often will my baby breastfeed? (feeding interval)

Frequent breastfeeding in the early weeks can have many benefits, by increasing your breasts' storage capacity, and perfecting your baby's feeding competence. Generally speaking, as a rule of thumb, feed your baby whenever he seems to want to go to the breast. Babies want to suck for comfort and entertainment as well as for hunger, and the breast can be your most effective mothering tool:

- A newborn may want to breastfeed at very short intervals as he learns how to hone his feeding skills.
- Most healthy babies want to breastfeed between 8 and 20 times in 24 hours, depending on
  > The baby's competence.
  > The mother's breast storage capacity (which is not necessarily related to the size of the breasts – breastfeeding very often in the first few weeks increases the mother's storage capacity, so that intervals may be longer later).

- If your baby is 'demanding', feed him on demand.
- As he obtains increasing quantities of milk, he may go longer between breastfeeds
- Most babies want to feed at *irregular* intervals, usually with longer feeding intervals in the mornings, and shorter intervals in the late afternoons and evenings.
- Many babies past the newborn stage cluster-feed in the evenings for several hours. Failure to go along with this can result in the baby becoming frantic, and this may be misnamed 'colic'.
- Babies who are allowed to cluster-feed in the late afternoon/ evening, usually eventually fall asleep and stay asleep for a longer 5–6 hour interval at night, from about 10pm to 3–4am. Over time these babies may take longer and longer sleeps at night.
- However, if your young baby seems sleepy, sleeping several periods of 3–5 hours in each 24 hour period, this is not a sign that he is getting enough. Sometimes we call these babies 'happy to starve' – he may not be getting enough milk to have the energy to be demanding (see Chapter 13). You will have to take control: wake him up to feed *at least* every three hours, day and night (three-hourly means from the start of one feed, to the start of the next).
- If your baby becomes very lethargic, and especially if he becomes jaundiced, start expressing/pumping your milk and feed it to your baby in another way (see Chapter 13).

Inadequate drainage

When the breasts become overfull or engorged, there can be several causes, as explained in Chapter 5, but the implications for HIV transmission remain the same. If the situation is not remedied quickly, it can lead to a cascade of negative effects. Tight junctions between the milk-producing cells can become damaged. Overfullness thus poses a risk for elevated viral levels and an increased risk of postnatal transmission of HIV.[6-8]

Special application of breast care for HIV-infected mothers

While *all* mothers should be provided with the knowledge and techniques they need to take care of their breasts and manage their own breastmilk supply, there are three special considerations that mothers living with HIV need to be aware of so that they can protect their babies:

- Breast engorgement (when the breasts become very full of milk) is a risk factor for increased breast permeability, and increased viral levels in breastmilk
- A compromised immune system makes a mother with HIV more at risk for a breast infection (mastitis)
- Unrelieved engorgement may reduce the breasts' storage capacity, compromising a mother's ability to exclusively breastfeed her baby for a full six months.[9]

Special care as the milk comes in – days 4–9 after birth

One of the most unfortunate pieces of advice that new mothers often receive is the old wives' tale *not* to drain very full breasts in the misconception that expressing or pumping will stimulate the breasts to make even more milk. It's not possible to over-emphasise that this is *not true*; it's likely based on a misunderstanding of the normal physiology of lactation. In fact, nothing will stop milk being produced as the milk 'comes in', since it is under what is called *endocrine control*. The time-lag in breast response means that overfull breasts can become even more overfull (engorged) very quickly and still more milk keeps being produced.

Thus it commonly happens that the mother's milk production temporarily outstrips the baby's appetite and a newborn baby doesn't take all the milk that the mother is making. For instance, on the fourth day of life, we would expect a 3kg baby to take about 450ml of breastmilk in 24 hours, whereas the mother may be making about 600ml. It takes several days for the baby's appetite to catch up with milk production so that they match. Meanwhile, if the breasts are not drained and engorgement is not resolved promptly it lays the groundwork for inadequate milk production later – the second most common reason for mothers to start formula-feeding (see Chapter 14).

If a mother follows advice not to express the extra milk it can trigger a truly calamitous situation,[10] especially in the context of HIV:

- as the baby leaves milk behind in the breasts, engorgement is exacerbated
- HIV levels in the milk rise as tight junctions in the breast are disrupted
- the breasts become hard, wooden, shiny and taut
- as engorgement worsens, the breasts become very difficult to express/pump
- a newborn can find latching to a hard, overfull breast difficult or impossible
- the worsening engorgement causes the milk-producing cells to flatten one against the other and they may burst. Whole lobes of breast tissue can become non-functional for that lactation. As the baby's appetite increases in the second week the mother finds that her milk production has dropped below her baby's needs; the baby needs to be fed, and will eventually require supplements of other milk
- breastfeeding + formula-feeding = mixed feeding
- mixed feeding is a risk factor for HIV transmission, requiring stopping breastfeeding.

The domino effect of lactation failure as described above is the second most common cause of breastfeeding failure, and is the root cause of 'not enough milk'.

Lactation management as preventive care

Importantly, these problems can be avoided. Preventive care is best. The mother herself can 'manage' her own breastmilk production. For a mother living with HIV, who needs to exclusively breastfeed for six full months, and for whom topping up with a bottle of formula if the baby is hungry later is not safe, there are several aspects she needs to consider. Taking care of over-fullness at this time will:

- protect her milk-producing cells from damage
- increase the number of prolactin receptors in the breast so that she continues to make plenty of milk into the later months when prolactin levels naturally fall to lower levels
- maximise the breast storage capacity
- reduce the risk of mastitis in the next few weeks (the time of greatest risk being 10 days–3 weeks, as a consequence of over-fullness in the previous few days)
- keep her baby growing and thriving with good weight gain on exclusive breastfeeding for six full months.

Preventing and addressing breast over-fullness promptly

Mothers can be warned about what will happen, and be given information about how to manage potential postpartum engorgement, as follows:

1. Breastfeed the baby as soon as possible after birth.
2. Breastfeed the 'demanding' baby in the first few days, for as long as he wants. Whenever the breasts start to feel even slightly too full, rouse the baby to breastfeed again.
3. However, if your baby is sleepy, wake him to feed and ensure that he breastfeeds at least eight and preferably 10–12 times in 24 hours.
4. Use rousing techniques to wake him
    > dab a cold wash-cloth on his face, or
    > undress him and change his nappy, or
    > place him alone on a hard surface until he realises he's alone.
5. Make sure the baby is able to attach easily and that breastfeeding is comfortable. Ask for help with positioning and attaching the baby to the breast if

> The baby is difficult to latch
> You feel pain, or if there is any damage to the nipple.
6. Ensure that the baby is breastfeeding with swallowing (he takes long slow sucks while the jaw drops, and pauses for swallowing in sucking bursts of 10 or so swallows), followed by a small rest, and then more swallowing.
7. Your full breasts should feel softer after feeding, showing that milk transfer (from you to the baby) has taken place.
8. The lactating breast normally has a cobblestone feel, but occasionally there can be areas which become overfull and you should pay attention to any hard lumpy areas, gently massaging them towards the nipple and feeding the baby again, or pumping until the whole breast feels reasonably soft and comfortable. If your breast is pretty well drained, the areola should feel as soft as your earlobe. If it is as hard as the tip of your nose, it is too full and you should try and feed the baby again, or express *more* milk.
9. Milk transfer/drainage (from the breasts to the baby) can also be assisted by 'breast compression'; when the baby takes a little pause between sucking bursts, gently compress the breast, being careful not to disturb the baby's latch (i.e. do not pull the nipple out of the baby's mouth), and then watch for the baby's swallowing again. Keep the breast still while the baby drinks, but use breast compression again at the next sucking pause.
10. Express or feed the baby whenever the breasts feel even a little too full from day 4–9, even if this is very often. It is very important to keep the breasts soft and comfortable and well-drained.
11. If the baby is too sleepy to breastfeed, hand-express or pump your milk so that he can be fed by cup or spoon (see Chapter 10).
12. Cabbage seems to act as a lactation suppressant; in between expressing you can tuck cool cabbage leaves around the breasts inside a T-shirt or a bra, to help to slow down breastmilk production:
    > wash and dry the leaves of a white cabbage and keep them

> in a clean plastic bag in the fridge
> tuck clean leaves around the breasts and change them every couple of hours
> *stop* using the cabbage as soon as your breasts seem to be making milk at the right rate for your baby, i.e. don't use them for so long that you don't have enough milk
13. After day 10, it is usual for:
    > The baby's appetite to have caught up with the mother's milk production
    > The breasts to have stopped feeling over-full.
14. Eventually your baby will begin to take all the milk you're making and you'll reach a state of equilibrium whereby you make enough milk for your baby's growing appetite and no longer need to express.
15. By day 14, most mothers find that their breasts are much softer and they may worry at this point that their milk has 'disappeared'. This is usually not the case – if you've been diligent about taking care of any engorgement, and if your baby has regained his birthweight and is producing adequate wet and dirty nappies, it just means that the baby is breastfeeding well and taking the milk you're making.
16. Thereafter, if the baby is taking enough, he should be fed 'on demand' (as often as he wants, for as long as he wants, but continue to pump/express if you need to any time you feel too full as described in Chapter 12).
17. Meanwhile you will have been protecting your breast tissue from irreversible damage, maximising your future breast storage capacity and setting the scene for being able to breastfeed exclusively for the next full six months.

If the milk fails to come in

If there is *not* a large increase in breastmilk production within at least the first five days after birth, then you should seek urgent medical advice from your healthcare team, because it points to a potentially serious medical problem (see Chapter 13). A common cause of delayed lactation, occurring in 1–3% of births, can be retained placental fragments which continue to secrete progesterone, hindering Lactogenesis II. This can be diagnosed by an ultrasound scan and can be treated by readmission to hospital for a D&C (dilation and curettage).[11] The milk will come in as normal after all the retained fragments have been removed. You need to seek prompt medical advice since retained placenta is a risk factor for a uterine infection or haemorrhage. Don't leave it!

Increasing breastmilk production in the first month

For a mother who is planning, for clear health reasons, to practise exclusive breastfeeding for the first six months of life, knowing how to 'manage' her breastmilk production to ensure enough milk for that length of time is important:

- the investment of time in breast care as the milk comes in and during the first month makes breastfeeding later so much easier
- frequent prolactin release that occurs with nipple stimulation (i.e. the baby sucking, or during pumping) acts on the milk-producing cells to make more milk for the next breastfeed,[12] increasing milk production over time
- high prolactin levels in early lactation also increase the number of prolactin receptor sites within the breast. When prolactin levels fall in later lactation, a larger number of receptor sites continue to respond to reducing levels of prolactin, so maintaining adequate lactation
- ensuring that the milk-producing cells within the breast remain intact and undamaged in the first two weeks maximises the breasts' storage capacity for later, potentially enabling the baby to obtain a larger quantity of milk at each breastfeed and to reduce the number of breastfeeds he takes in 24 hours.[9]

Ongoing milk production and fluctuations in supply

All being well, and building on the care taken during the first two weeks, breastmilk production continues to go up and up during the first month after birth. Most thriving babies will take 750–900ml in 24 hours and research shows that from 1–6 months that amount doesn't increase.[13]

Breastmilk synthesis is a dynamic process. As long as the breasts are well drained, then they will go on producing milk. To increase milk production, the baby may indicate that he wants to breastfeed more often, and if he's responded to for a few days, the breasts will begin to make more milk. If the breasts are consistently drained very well then they start to produce a little more milk, and sooner, and then even more, even sooner.

Breastfeeding on demand

In later weeks, breast tissue continues to be extremely responsive to the degree of fullness in the milk-producing cells. If not drained out of the breasts certain proteins in the milk (called feedback inhibitor of lactation, FIL) signal the milk-producing cells to make less. If they are consistently kept a little too full, then they start to produce a little less and then even less and to fill more slowly.

Test-expressing after feeding can indicate to the mother how effectively her baby has breastfed; if she is able to express jets of milk after breastfeeding, then this shows that the baby has not drained the breast well. If she is only able to express creamy drops, then this is an indication that the breast is well drained.

A mother who has successfully navigated the first few weeks of the learning period, so that her baby is healthy, thriving and gaining weight well, and wants to be sure of making enough milk for the full recommended time of six months' exclusive breastfeeding, should breastfeed her baby:

- whenever he wants
- for as long as he wants
- at irregular intervals, usually 10–12 times in 24 hours
- ensuring that he takes only one 4–5 hour sleep in 24 hours (newborns may take this in the morning, older babies may start sleeping longer at night).

The mother with a low storage capacity in her breasts may find that she really needs to feed her baby 20 times in 24 hours. In addition, most breastfed babies don't feed at set intervals – they may cluster-feed (5–6 times) over the space of 2–3 hours and then sleep for a couple of hours and then wake for another cluster-feed.

Urine/stool output

The baby's urine and stool output can provide a way to monitor from day to day that the baby is getting enough breastmilk. A healthy, thriving baby should produce:

- *Day 1:* 1 wet nappy, black meconium stool
- *Day 2:* 2 wet nappies, brown stool
- *Day 3:* 3 wet nappies, 1–2 changing stools
- *Day 4:* 4 wet nappies, 1–2 brown-yellow stools
- *Day 5:* 5 wet nappies, 2–3 yellow seedy stools
- *From the first week:* 6–8 wet cloth or five heavy disposable nappies (clear urine) and 3–5 yellow, seedy stools in each 24 hours

Baby's weight

Weighing your baby frequently in the beginning can help to reassure you that your baby is 'getting enough'. A healthy, thriving baby who is breastfeeding effectively usually doubles his birthweight in 3–5 months, and meanwhile meets the following goals at the following times:

- *3 days:* loss of not more than 7% of his birthweight
- *10–14 days:* regains birthweight
- *3 days–3 months:* has an average gain of 30g/day (210g/week)
- *3 months–6 months:* has an average gain of 20g/day (140g/week)

Taking your baby for weighing on a regular basis, especially in the early weeks, and plotting his weight on a chart (eg the World Health Organization chart[14]) can:

- reassure you that he is gaining well, or
- give you an early warning if his rate of gain is starting to slow down so that you can remedy the situation/change something
- allow you to see if he is following an adequate growth curve along the percentile on which he was born.

Enlist the cooperation of your local clinic or health visitor so that you can have weight checks done:

- weekly for the first six weeks
- fortnightly for a couple of months
- monthly until six months

You'll be very proud to see your baby growing and thriving exclusively on your milk.

If the baby who has been breastfeeding well suddenly seems to be unhappy and more demanding, it is worth checking his weight and comparing it with the above guidelines. The weights always tell a story and help you work out if there's a problem or not:

- If the baby's weight gain is a bit low, it can be worthwhile breastfeeding more often for several days to see if he becomes more content, and then weighing again to make sure he is gaining well.
- perhaps the mother has started hormonal birth control, or another medication which suppresses lactation somewhat, or there may have been a change in the sleeping/eating pattern.
- If the baby is gaining well but is still unhappy, he may be showing a sensitivity to a particular food in the mother's diet.
- If the baby is breastfeeding often but not gaining well, then review suggestions in Chapter 14 to increase his intake, and seek medical advice to rule out an infection.
- If the baby seems unhappy and is not gaining weight well, it might be worth consulting your IBCLC or breastfeeding counsellor for possible causes and suggestions to resolve low

gain or a dwindling milk supply. There is also more information in Chapter 14. There is usually a cause that can be identified, and a care plan can be developed to resolve the problem.

Sleeping patterns

The 'demanding' healthy baby's own feeding and sleeping pattern should be trusted. It is damaging to continued breastmilk production to try and impose any kind of sleeping programme on a breastfed baby (e.g. lengthening feeding intervals by leaving the baby to cry in the hope that he will sleep longer). Most newborns are more wakeful and hungry at night than they are in the day, and this works to increase breastmilk synthesis because the mother's prolactin levels are higher at night too. If the mother responds to the baby's need to feed, most older babies will eventually start to take their longest sleep at night (often from about 10pm to 3 or 4am), and this long interval may extend to even six or seven hours. The baby can be described as 'sleeping through the night' if he sleeps for six hours.

When a baby is sleeping too long to breastfeed often enough, and failing to gain adequate weight, then the mother needs to take charge and wake him up to feed more often (see Chapter 13).

Mothering the mother

Arranging your life so that you can make this special but challenging time as easy as possible for yourself is well worthwhile (review the suggestions at the end of Chapter 3). The more time you invest early on, the easier you will find breastfeeding later.

8. MIXED BREASTFEEDING AFTER SIX MONTHS

Mothers living with HIV who have chosen to exclusively breastfeed their babies for the first half-year are increasingly opting to continue breastfeeding past the six-month mark when their babies start receiving solid foods. Is this safe?

Technically, once the baby is fed anything else as well as breastmilk, it would be described as 'mixed breastfeeding'. Mixed breastfeeding *before six months* is shown to be a risk factor for HIV transmission. Damage and inflammation in the infant's immature gut caused by other foods and liquids can more easily allow transmission of any virus in breastmilk to come into contact with the baby's bloodstream (see Chapter 5). Thus the fear that breastfeeding after six months is a risk factor for HIV transmission underpins the suggestion for early weaning.

Is advice to stop breastfeeding at six months still valid?

However, the baby *older than six months* has a mature gastrointestinal tract and the situation is entirely different from other foods and liquids being given to a baby younger than six months. Crucially, when the baby has been exclusively breastfed for the first half-year, breastmilk is able to contribute to maturation of the gut.[1] The exclusively breastfed baby reaches six months with an intact intestinal mucosa, and when the mother continues to be meticulously adherent to her ART, the risk of transmission of HIV is probably negligible (see Chapter 3).

Research from Zambia and Tanzania confirmed that the babies of mothers receiving ART showed very low rates of HIV infection at six and 12 months.[2] There were *no* transmissions at all through breastfeeding when mothers had a very low viral load. The only transmissions during mixed breastfeeding after six months occurred in women who were non-adherent to their medications.[3]

In the UK, mothers living with HIV enjoy an even better prognosis, since they have usually received ART from before or during very early pregnancy, which is continued for life, leading to an undetectable viral load by the time of birth (when breastfeeding begins).

A 2013 paper written by a WHO Interagency Task Team concluded that the risk of HIV transmission decreases as a child's gut matures, and that mixed feeding does not carry the same risk after the age of six months.[4] This is because breastmilk contains growth factors which help to mature the gut lining, and hinder passage of the virus. Also, antiretroviral drugs have shifted the risk/benefit analysis in favour of breastfeeding. Several trials have demonstrated that mothers with HIV can breastfeed safely for longer durations. The best available evidence suggests that the risk to the baby from other diseases if breastfeeding stops before the age of one are greater than the potential side-effects of prolonged drug exposure. The WHO Team suggests that when mothers decide to stop breastfeeding, weaning should be done gradually, within one month. Weaning abruptly is not advisable because it is associated with mastitis and elevated viral load in breastmilk.

The British HIV Association guidance[5] points to global recommendations developed by the World Health Organization in 2016,[6] which make no distinction in breastfeeding recommendations depending on whether a mother has HIV or not. Both inside and outside the context of HIV, exclusive breastfeeding is recommended for the first six months of life, followed by continued breastfeeding with household weaning foods for up to 12–24 months.

Why carry on past six months?

The World Health Organization suggests that around the age of six months, an infant's need for energy and nutrients starts to exceed what breastmilk alone can provide, but even in the context of HIV WHO guidance advises mothers to breastfeed for up to two years or beyond. Solid foods would be an addition to, not a replacement for, breastmilk at first.

The baby is developmentally ready for other foods when:

- He shows an interest in what the rest of the family is eating
- He can grab things and take them to his mouth
- He can sit up
- His tongue protrusion reflex has resolved. When offered a mouthful of food, immature babies who are too young for solid foods will push it out on to the chin where the mother has to scrape it up and offer the food again; babies who are developmentally ready for solids will take the food to the back of the tongue and swallow it.

If your baby has fulfilled all these criteria, then WHO recommends[7] that his growth may falter if he does not receive complementary foods. Foods in addition to breastmilk should be:

- *Timely* – meaning that they are introduced when the need for energy and nutrients exceeds what can be provided through exclusive breastfeeding;
- *Adequate* – meaning that they provide sufficient energy, protein and micronutrients to meet a growing child's nutritional needs;
- *Safe* – meaning that they are hygienically stored and prepared, and fed with clean hands using clean utensils and not bottles and teats;
- *Properly fed* – meaning that they are given according to a child's signals of appetite and satiety, and that meal frequency and feeding are suitable for age.
- *Young children should usually receive three main meals plus two snacks in 24 hours.*
- Caregivers should take active care in the feeding of infants by being responsive to the child's cues for hunger and also encouraging the child to eat.

Mothers with HIV who have succeeded in breastfeeding exclusively for the first six months of their baby's life are usually well aware of the convenience of breastfeeding and of its importance in their relationship with the baby. It is often much easier to carry on breastfeeding than to stop, and there are real nutritional, emotional and immunological reasons for continuing.

Nutritional advantages

Once the older baby starts taking increasing quantities of other foods, the nutrition provided by breastmilk may seem to be less valuable. However, spoonful for spoonful, breastmilk contains more calories than many weaning foods. In addition, breastmilk contains components which act separately and in combination as an advantage to the baby, and is more than the sum of its parts.[8] Breastmilk is brain food; it contributes to optimal cognitive development.[9] Breastmilk can still also provide the following proportion of the older baby's nutritional needs:

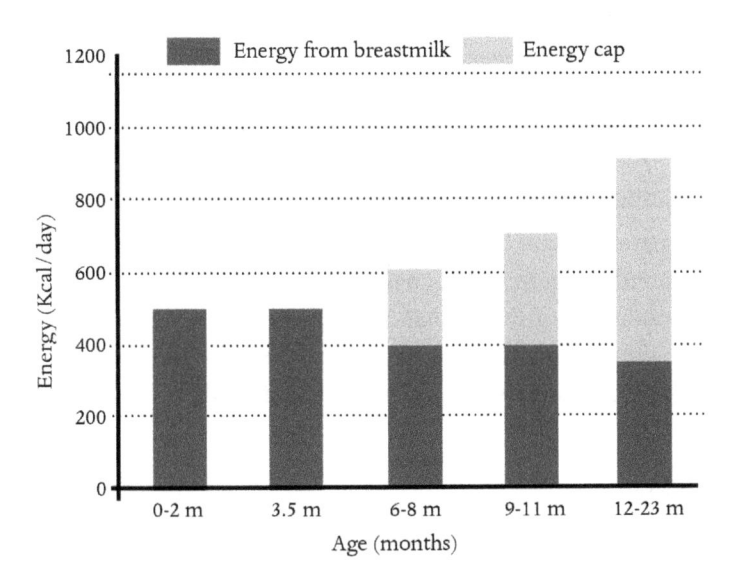

Adapted from World Health Organization (2009). Infant and young child feeding: model chapter for textbooks for medical students and allied health professionals. https://pubmed.ncbi.nlm.nih.gov/23905206/

Immunological considerations

Breastfeeding after six months provides important immunological benefits to the older baby. As normal weaning progresses, the immunological components in a lower volume of breastmilk become more concentrated so that even a small quantity every day provides an important means of protection against disease. A still-breastfeeding toddler will remain healthier than one who is already weaned.[10-13]

Emotional benefits

It has been well recognised by the breastfeeding support organisations such as La Leche League that breastfeeding means a whole lot more than just food to both mother and baby.[14] A mother who is still breastfeeding can always comfort and console her baby, or calm a sick child at the breast and help him to fall asleep very easily in a way that no other mothering skills can quite match. Thus the emotional benefits of breastfeeding begin to assume greater importance for the mother of an older baby. In addition, cultural practices for many mothers living with HIV favour continued breastfeeding into toddlerhood.[15]

Discuss breastfeeding past six months with your multi-disciplinary team

All these matters need to be taken into consideration. Clearly babies over six months require additional food, but does this addition require weaning from the breast? Mothers living with HIV who wish to continue breastfeeding beyond six months should have further meetings to discuss their plans with their multi-disciplinary team (MDT).

Cases in the UK

Can your MDT obtain more information about other mothers living with HIV who have breastfed? What is the rate of HIV transmission through breastfeeding when 'ideal scenario' conditions are fulfilled?

- Mothers have received ART for several months before the birth

- There has been strict adherence to ART
- Mother has an undetectable viral load
- The baby has been exclusively breastfeeding for the first half-year

The July 2021 ISOSS Report includes records for babies who had been breastfed for periods ranging from one day to two years.[16] At a webinar to disseminate the results of the UK NOURISH study, held on 19 October 2022, it was reported that not one of these babies had been infected with HIV.

Continuing to breastfeed safely

If you're a mother with HIV who decides to breastfeed after six months you should:

- continue meticulous ART adherence
- continue attending viral load testing appointments
- continue taking your baby for HIV testing at recommended times
- keep follow-up appointments with your HIV clinicians, and your baby's paediatrician
- take immediate measures to pump or express your milk to avoid the breasts becoming overfull if there should be any sudden changes in your baby's breastfeeding pattern, e.g. lengthening breastfeeding intervals by sleeping through the night, mother-baby separation due to social events or work (see Chapter 7, breastmilk production and Chapter 9 on weaning)
- seek medical advice if you experience any breast or nipple problems, and follow the recommendations for self-care set out in chapters 12 and 13
- follow the baby's lead about what and how much other food he will accept. Proceed carefully in trusting his willingness to accept various foods so as to avoid food sensitivities; these are unlikely if the baby has been exclusively breastfed for six months, but should be respected.[17]

Caution: risk of HIV transmission with pre-chewed food

Whether to offer pureed or mashed foods (as recommended by WHO and the NHS) or to offer whole foods (termed baby-led weaning) is a matter of individual choice.[18] However, traditional methods of feeding babies and toddlers in some parts of the world have involved a mother, grandmother or other carer using pre-chewed/pre-masticated foods, to soften weaning foods and make them more digestible. Saliva from an infected carer can pass HIV to the weanling and this practice has been identified in recent years as a route of HIV transmission.[19] It's therefore recommended that mothers do not use pre-chewing as a method of feeding their babies solid foods, and that they use caution about what is being fed to the baby by others.

9. WEANING FROM THE BREAST

In 2016 the World Health Organization revised its HIV and infant feeding guidance to recommend that in the context of HIV babies should be exclusively breastfed for six months and continue breastfeeding for up to 24 months.[1] In other words, their recommendations did not differ based on whether or not a mother was living with HIV.

Definition of weaning

Weaning has a double meaning in English:

- To introduce other foods and liquids into the breastfed baby's diet (to start solid foods)
- To stop breastfeeding completely

Weaning actually begins when the baby starts to receive any other foods or liquids besides breastmilk (as recommended for all babies from the middle of the first year) and is completed when the baby has received his last breastfeed. Weaning can be either:

- *mother-led:* the mother picks a date when she will no longer breastfeed, or
- *baby-led:* which is often so gradual that it can only be identified as the mother looks backwards and realises that, as the days go by, the baby no longer goes to the breast.

Anticipating weaning

For the mother living with HIV who has breastfed her baby successfully for many weeks or months, the thought of stopping breastfeeding can stir up some ambivalent feelings. When breastfeeding will have been an unusual and difficult achievement in a First World country where the common understanding is that if you have HIV you probably shouldn't have babies, let alone breastfeed them, she will feel proud that she has been able to breastfeed her baby. On the one hand, she may look forward to a time when there will be no further risk of mother-to-child transmission of the virus to her child. On the other hand she may have a sense of how she will miss breastfeeding her little one once he is weaned. She will also have an awareness of how much she depends on breastfeeding to enable her to mother her baby in any situation, and how breastfeeding has become a central pillar of their relationship. So there is a bitter-sweetness to contemplating weaning.

Preparing for weaning

The major considerations are:

- To augment the baby's diet after six months, so that he starts to receive other foods, particularly iron-containing foods like meat
- To slowly replace the nutrition that the baby currently receives from breastmilk with other foods and liquids (see Chapter 8)
- To find alternatives to sucking and comfort which are currently met at the breast, and that *are as acceptable to the baby as breastfeeding*
- To be aware of the return of fertility once breastfeeding ends
- To maintain the mother's breast health as the baby takes less milk. Weaning from the breast needs to be carefully managed by mothers with HIV because:
  > viral load in the breastmilk can rise if there is milk stasis (milk undrained from the breast)
  > there is an increased risk of mastitis if the breasts remain undrained.

The baby's nutrition

There are many resources giving ideas about how to add solid foods to your baby's diet.[2,3] After six months, you're working towards your baby starting to eat the same foods as the rest of the family. As he takes less and less breastmilk, the mother can offer smooth purees, then mashed or chopped foods, and eventually foods that he can chew. However, the nutrition provided by breastmilk can still continue to be important into the third year of life. See also Chapter 8.

Unless you absolutely have to wean quickly, abrupt weaning at any age can be dangerous. The baby may become inconsolable and is at risk for malnutrition or kwashiorkor if he becomes so distressed that he will not eat, nor take any other milk by bottle.[4]
In this case, before weaning from the breast altogether, it would be safer to continue breastfeeding for a little longer, in order to accustom him to receiving (your) milk by bottle, and then other milks and other foods.

The baby's emotional wellbeing

A baby under two years of age will have high sucking needs that are currently met through breastfeeding.[5] Will he accept a bottle-feed instead of a breastfeed? Will he take a dummy? Does he suck his thumb or fingers for comfort, or does he have another comfort object to fall asleep with? If the baby is already used to a bottle and alternative comfort objects before you start weaning, as set out in Chapter 4, then weaning will be easier than if the breast is his sole comfort object.

Friends and family may suggest harsh weaning methods such as leaving the baby to 'cry it out', or leaving him with the grandmother or an aunt for a week or two, but the baby will be able to accept weaning from the breast more easily if he only has to deal with the loss of the breast rather than the loss of his mother as well. The mother anticipating the loss of breastfeeding may like to save some mementoes, such as arranging a breastfeeding photo-shoot, or buying some breastmilk jewellery, as a way to honour and remember this very special relationship.

How does the baby go to sleep?

When weaning from the breast, and especially if the baby is used to nursing to sleep, you may need to introduce other comfort measures such as holding, patting or rocking. You may need to be inventive about thinking of alternatives to breastfeeding which the baby will accept, especially if he wakes up and nurses back to sleep several times in the night. Maybe you can use other comfort measures during naptimes at first and when these are acceptable then use them for night-time too. Maybe the baby's father can help rock the baby to sleep, but some babies indicate a definite preference for the mother, and having a plan in advance will make weaning easier.

Breastfeeding and contraception – your fertility

Exclusive breastfeeding for up to six months is known to provide 98% protection against another pregnancy. This is more effective than the progestin-only pill. However, the contraceptive effect of breastfeeding is only effective when all three of the following conditions are met:[6]

- The mother's periods have not yet returned after the birth
- The baby is breastfeeding around the clock and doesn't sleep for longer than six hours at night
- The baby is under six months of age.

This means that as soon as you start weaning your baby from the breast, your fertility can return. Unless you are planning another pregnancy, it might be a good idea to seek advice on contraception. Conversely, some women find that their periods do not return while they are still breastfeeding, and they may not ovulate until their baby is a year of age or more. If they want to have another baby, they may decide to wean for this reason.

How easy is it to wean?

Weaning a happily breastfeeding baby from the breast is not easy. Ironically, the more challenging it is, the more of a testament that is to the success of the breastfeeding relationship.

Mothers describe many ambivalent feelings:

- the older the baby, the harder it is
- weaning for clear medical reasons seems to be easier because there is a firm rationale for it
- the less committed the mother feels to the need for weaning, the more difficult it may seem
- as the baby enters toddlerhood, the emotional benefits of breastfeeding often come to mean more to the mother and child, and the nutritional aspects seem less important
- there can be real sadness and grief, often unrecognised by family, friends or even a mother's clinicians, though weaning grief is a real phenomenon, long recognised by breastfeeding counsellors and IBCLCs.[7]

Practical weaning strategies
- Offer other foods and liquids, or a bottle of infant formula, to replace one breastfeed every few days (see Chapter 8)
- Monitor your child's urine and stool output, and his weight to ensure that he continues to get enough to eat; the weaning child will stop producing the yellow seedy stools of the breastfed baby, and the stools should become firmer as he takes more other adult foods
- Toddlers often ask to breastfeed much more often if they are developing very fast in another area, e.g. learning to walk, learning to talk, becoming more sociable; or if there is a change in their lives, e.g. going on holiday, if friends and relations are visiting, mother starting work, child going to a new playgroup or childminder, etc. It may be harder to wean during these times
- Babies often breastfeed for entertainment or because they are bored, as well as for comfort; mothers who want to wean may need to become very inventive, change their normal routine and use a lot of distraction *before* the baby asks to breastfeed
- Set limits; instead of being willing to breastfeed anytime, anywhere, start having only one place where you will breastfeed, somewhere away from the TV, other people etc.

The child then has to stop what he's doing to access the breast, i.e. he can't multi-task, or breastfeed while doing something else. Eventually he will stop asking to breastfeed every time you sit down in your favourite chair
- Wear clothes that make it difficult for the baby to help himself to the breast
- Some mothers adopt a 'never offer, never refuse' strategy – you may relax this if your baby becomes sick, and start limiting breastfeeding again when he recovers
- Provide lots of 'other mothering'; lots of cuddles and carrying, one-to-one attention, stories, and games so that your baby knows he still has your attention, even if he doesn't breastfeed as much as he did before
- Be prepared to be flexible. If your baby's behaviour deteriorates and you find he is becoming clingy and throwing tantrums, you may need to proceed more slowly. If he seems to be handling fewer breastfeeds per day you can go faster
- Babies vary in which breastfeeds they will give up last; for some it's the bedtime feed; for others it may be the early-morning breastfeed after they wake up
- Even after official weaning, you may find that you want to continue to breastfeed for comfort after bumps, falls, during an illness or a crisis.

Slowing down milk production

It is important never to leave the breasts to become too full. Mothers don't always realise how much milk they're making:

- An exclusively breastfed baby coming up to six months will usually be taking about 850–900ml of breastmilk in each 24 hours
- Between six and 12 months a partially breastfed baby will usually be taking about 500ml of breastmilk each day.

Active mother-led weaning if the baby is under six months

- If you haven't already accustomed your baby to taking your expressed breastmilk by bottle (see chapters 3 and 5), start weaning by teaching your baby to take *your own milk* in a bottle. Offer small amounts often, reward the baby with big smiles and proceed slowly until you feel confident that he is able to take a bottle easily.
- Start weaning by replacing one breastmilk-feeding a day with a bottle of infant formula. *To avoid mixed feeding you will have to immediately stop all breastfeeding,* and instead express/pump your breasts and pasteurise your expressed breastmilk before feeding it to the baby (see Chapter 11).
- Every few days replace another bottle of breastmilk with a bottle of formula so that he is taking two formula-feeds each day, and then three, and so on until you have replaced all breastmilk-feeds and the baby is completely formula-fed.
- It's important not to allow the breasts to become over-full or engorged. Express whenever you feel more than just a little too full.
- The milk should be pasteurised before storing, or after storing.
- You can save the milk in the fridge or freezer to feed by bottle at another time, but if your baby is younger than six months any breastmilk fed to a baby who is also receiving formula should be pasteurised.

If you are weaning very fast

For the HIV+ mother, rapid weaning is specifically not recommended,[8] due to:

- increased risk of infections and mortality in the baby
- breast overfullness that can lead to opening of tight junctions in the breast, to allow elevated viral levels in the milk, posing an increased risk of HIV transmission to the baby
- risks to the mother's health, especially an increased risk of mastitis.

The mother has the option of expressing the breasts for comfort, pasteurising the expressed breastmilk and bottle-feeding it to the baby as described in Chapter 13; this avoids mixing raw breastmilk and other foods or formula in the baby's gut.

Rapid weaning needs very careful breast care/lactation management:

- express only as much milk as you need in order to keep the breasts comfortable
- express as often as you need to
- gradually the intervals between needing to express will lengthen
- gradually the amount of milk you need to express will reduce
- use cabbage leaves inside the bra to hasten suppression of lactation (see Chapter 7)
- do not bind the breasts
- do not limit fluids; drink to thirst
- wear a loose soft bra or T-shirt to provide breast support without increasing tension within the breasts
- a baby under 12 months should receive formula to replace breastmilk
- a baby over 12 months can receive cow's milk instead of breastmilk

Slow weaning

In the context of HIV the slower and more gently the breasts stop producing milk, the safer it will be for the baby and the more comfortable it will be for the mother.

If at all possible, it is always less risky to both mother and baby to suppress lactation in the most gradual way possible, allowing both mother and baby to absorb the physical consequences of not breastfeeding, and – if necessary – allowing the possibility of reversing this decision should something unexpected occur.

Breast size and shape

Mothers often worry about the consequences of breastfeeding on the breasts, and particularly if the breasts will sag after weaning. It is pregnancy, not breastfeeding, which exerts the major effect on the breasts. During pregnancy, some of the fatty tissue in the breasts is replaced by milk-producing cells. During slow weaning the milk-producing tissue gradually involutes or shrinks as the fat in the breasts is gradually replaced. It takes about six weeks after stopping breastfeeding altogether for the breasts to stop producing milk, and some women who have breastfed for a long time find that it takes much longer than that.[9]

Shortly after weaning is completed, the breasts may seem to be 'empty' and softer and smaller than during breastfeeding. Saggy breasts are more likely with rapid weaning, though this is temporary. Gradual weaning is kinder on the breasts since it allows more time for fat to be laid down to replace the involuting milk-making cells. As stressed so often, engorgement is very damaging to the breasts and should be avoided (see suggestions in Chapter 7). With each menstrual cycle following weaning, your breasts will start to firm up and gradually resume their normal shape and size, though after you have had a baby they may always be a little softer.

10. EXPRESSING, PUMPING, STORING AND FEEDING BREASTMILK

Mothers living with HIV who are planning to exclusively breastfeed their babies for the first six months of life should nevertheless know how to breastmilk-feed as a back-up feeding method if something unexpected happens.

Many mothers feed their expressed breastmilk to their babies, rather than breastfeeding direct, for a short time or a long time. Breastmilk-feeding can be undertaken by necessity, to feed the baby, or it may be the mother's choice, for a variety of reasons.

Breastmilk-feeding can be useful in several different situations:

- From choice; a mother may want her baby to receive her own milk, but she may not want to put the baby to the breast. Such a mother will express or pump her milk, put it in a bottle and exclusively breastmilk-feed by bottle for as long as she wants. Breastmilk-feeding is possible for weeks, months or even years, and there is no particular age that the baby doesn't really need her milk any more. The World Health Organization recommends exclusive breastfeeding for the first six months of life (nothing but breastmilk) and partial breastfeeding (with the addition of other foods and liquids) for up to two years or beyond.[1] Breastmilk-feeding can follow the same course.
- From necessity for a few days, if the baby is having difficulty latching, or is actually refusing the breast. If this happens you can hand-express your milk and feed it to the baby by another route (cup, spoon or bottle).
- To 'rest' sore nipples. You can express or pump your milk to feed the baby for a few days, without nursing the baby direct at the breast, so that the nipples can heal. When returning to breastfeeding direct again, you can rest the nipples for every other feed and breastfeed for every other feed, or every two

feeds, as a way to ease back into breastfeeding direct.
- To avoid breastfeeding direct during an episode of mastitis. The affected breast should be very well drained in order to assist resolution of the infection, and the expressed breastmilk can be flash-heated to inactivate any elevated levels of virus in the milk (see Chapter 11). Once all symptoms (pain, inflammation, indurated areas) have resolved then breastfeeding direct can be resumed.
- To feed an older baby who is suddenly refusing the breast/on a nursing strike (see Chapter 14) until he can be persuaded to return to breastfeeding again. Express/pump the breasts often and feed enough breastmilk by bottle to keep the baby happy and well-fed and start implementing the strategies described in Chapter 14. If the strike is not over in 3–4 days, consider contacting your IBCLC as soon as possible for more help to resolve the strike.
- To provide expressed breastmilk for someone else to feed the baby occasionally, e.g. the father, other family members, if the mother has to be separated from the baby for work, school, or social events.

Hand-express or pump?

Different methods work more efficiently at different times, depending on breast fullness and the stage of lactation:

- When the breast is not very full, it works better to hand-express the breasts rather than pump:
  > E.g. for the first 2–3 days after the birth of your baby
  > Using fingers on your breast (skin on skin) is likely to trigger your let-down reflex to work more efficiently at first
  > When the amount of milk or colostrum to be expressed is scanty, you can catch more precious drops if you express into a small cup (like a medicine cup) or a spoon (for direct feeding to the baby)
  > Using a pump on a relatively 'empty' breast can mean that

more milk/colostrum is wasted on the sides of the flange than can be saved in a container and when every drop is precious, this makes a difference
  > Hand-expression seems to be more efficient on an empty breast, and a pump seems to work better on a full breast
  > The suction of a pump (designed to suck milk out of the breast) seems to be more uncomfortable when there is less milk
- When the breast is fairly full, (e.g. after your milk has come in from day 2–4) you will probably find that a pump works more efficiently to drain the breasts.
  > If you're using a double pump, it's quicker still
  > If you're finding that your let-down is slow to start, try hand-expressing for a minute or two, and then when your let-down is triggered, move to the pump
  > If you're trying to drain the breasts very well, it can work well to pump first and then hand-express the last few creamy drops.

How often to express

1. You can start expressing colostrum within a few hours of baby's birth if you need colostrum for a baby who is not latching.
2. Continue to express the breasts very thoroughly at least seven times in 24 hours (every three hours in the day, with perhaps one longer interval for sleep at night) to provide enough milk for the baby and to keep the breasts soft and comfortable.
3. Express the breasts more often if they become overfull – it is vital to continued long-term breastmilk production that the breasts are drained often enough (especially from day 4–9 postpartum) to avoid/resolve engorgement and prevent elevation of HIV levels in the milk.
4. Also express more often (even every 90 minutes) if inadequate milk is being produced; over time, very frequent and thorough drainage increases the rate of breastmilk synthesis and overall milk production.

5. Occasionally, mothers who are making too much milk in the newborn period will express the milk so that the breasts feel soft and comfortable, and then find that the baby wakes up and seems especially hungry. The lesson here is: do not discard any extra breastmilk expressed from the breasts. Store the extra in the usual way.
6. After day 10, ongoing breastmilk production is directly dependant on drainage of the breasts and the amount produced may fluctuate slightly from day to day.
7. Once lactation is very well established, mothers may be able to express as much as 250ml at each session, so a baby needing 750ml of milk in 24 hours would only require the mother to express 3–4 times in 24 hours. However, if there is a subsequent drop in milk production as a result of infrequent drainage of the breasts, you may need to express more often again for a few days, until the quantity produced returns to normal.

Storing breastmilk

1. Expressed breastmilk should be stored in covered containers, e.g. a jam-jar, or a bottle with a lid, or in commercially manufactured breastmilk storage bags. Always write the date on the container to create your own use-by dates.
2. Breastmilk may retain more nutrients if stored in brown glass, rather than clear glass, or if otherwise protected from light.
3. Sterilising:
   > If used for formula, bottles and teats should always be sterilised.
   > If used for a hospitalised baby, all equipment should also be sterilised.
   > If used for a full-term healthy baby at home, containers for storing breastmilk, and cups and spoons for feeding should be washed and clean, but need not be sterilised.
4. Raw breastmilk can be safely stored at the following temperatures, for the following lengths of time:[2]

> Room temperature, cool day: 6–8 hours
> Room temperature, hot day (> 25°C): six hours
> Refrigerator (4°C) : 5–8 days
> Freezer (-18°C): six months

5. Breastmilk which has been pasteurised may be safely stored in the fridge, or in a covered jar at room temperature for eight hours afterwards if the jar remains unopened (i.e. so long as the milk is not subsequently exposed to bacteria from hands or other containers).
6. For a full-term healthy baby, breastmilk in a sucked bottle or from a sucked cup need not be discarded. Leftover breastmilk can be refrigerated for 48 hours, rewarmed, and fed to baby at the next feed. However, it should not be reused more than once.[3]

The benefits to the baby of feeding a mother's own breastmilk

Compared to formula, mother's milk is:[4]

- Physiologically normal for her particular baby, i.e. it changes over time, and contains the right nutrients, human proteins, fats and sugars, enzymes and antibodies.
- Immunologically complete. The mother produces antibodies in her milk to bacteria and viruses to which both she and her baby are exposed.
- Nutritionally perfect for human babies.
- The normal maternal postpartum hormonal profile is maintained, which
  > promotes maternal-infant bonding
  > is likely to maintain lactational amenorrhea/reduce fertility
- Safe
- Free
- Feasible
- Within the mother's control, e.g. she safeguards the baby's milk supply/sustainability/baby's food security (important in emergencies and when away from home)

- Bottles which will be used for feeding breastmilk do not need to be sterilised after use (unlike bottles which will be used for formula)
- Especially advantageous for a second or subsequent baby who is
  > more at risk for sensitisation to cow's milk-based formula and thus more likely to suffer colic, asthma, eczema etc
  > exposed to more colds and other infections brought home by older siblings

How to hand express or pump

Hand expression is a learned skill. But it's like riding a bicycle; easy once you know how. Several organisations have posted videos on the internet of how to hand express.[5,6]

1. Wash your hands. It's not necessary to wash the breasts more often than once a day during your ordinary bath or shower.
2. It may help the milk to 'flow' if warm cloths or warm water are used on the breasts before pumping or expressing (including a warm shower or warm bath).
3. Massage the breast gently before starting to express the milk; use the fingertips or knuckles to gently knead the breast from the ribs in towards the nipples; this helps to move the milk from the back of the breasts down (or up) towards the areola/nipple. Always handle the breasts using light pressure; neither massage, nor hand-expression, should ever hurt. If it does, lighten the pressure.
4. Cup the breast with one hand, with fingers underneath and thumb on top. The pad of the index finger and thumb should be placed on or behind the areola about 2–3cm behind the nipple.
5. Using the whole hand to take the weight of the breast, press the thumb and first finger inwards directly towards the chest wall.
6. Then squeeze the thumb and forefinger gently together (this should not hurt!)
7. It may take a minute or two for your let-down to be triggered so be patient and keep gently expressing until you see milk, then

breastmilk will usually drip or squirt from the nipple pores.
8. Once your milk starts flowing, hold the squeeze until the milk stops dripping or squirting, then once the milk flow stops, release the pressure on the nipple/areola, and start again.
9. When one area of the breast seems to be drained and the milk stops flowing, move your fingers so that you cover different ducts. Imagine the breast is a clock-face – you could place finger and thumb at 12 and 6 o'clock, then move to 9 and 3 o'clock, then 8 and 2 o'clock and finally 10 and 4 o'clock.
10. If you are expressing the breasts one at a time, once all the ducts seem to be drained and the breast has stopped flowing, start expressing the other breast in the same way until the flow of milk stops.
11. If necessary, massage and express the first breast a second time, and the second breast a second time.
12. Continue expressing until sufficient milk has been drained from each breast that both are soft and comfortable.
13. To save time, you can hand-express both breasts simultaneously, by using two hands and balancing a collection bowl on a pillow on your lap.

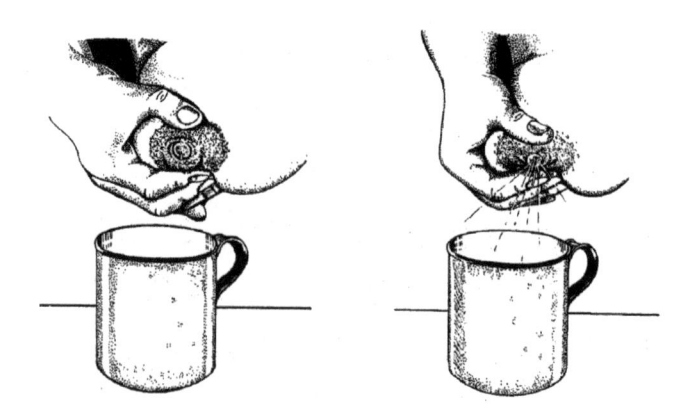

WHO HIV & Infant Feeding Counselling Course, 2000 [7]

Using a breast pump

Some mothers prefer to use a pump, rather than hand express. Pumps vary in quality and some work better than others. The most efficient is a double electric hospital-grade pump and the investment you make in arranging access to one during the newborn period will give you a good return many times over. Some companies will hire out pumps and deliver them to your door within 24 hours and it might be worth booking this as soon as your baby is born so that you're prepared for the first two weeks.

- Expect your pump to exert quite a strong suck. When the nipple and areola are centred in the flange of the pump and you start pumping, the nipple should be drawn into the flange, to be released when suction is reversed. If this doesn't happen, seek help quickly: the fault is more likely to be with the pump than with the mother.
- Pumps often have different sucking modes. You need a quick low-suction action for a couple of minutes to trigger your let-down reflex, and then a slow higher-suction mode when the milk starts flowing. Some pumps have been designed to make this switch automatically as a result of research into what works to maximise milk yield. Set the suction to your own comfort level – it should draw the nipple and some of the areola into the flange, but it shouldn't suck so hard that it's uncomfortable.
- Milk should start to flow from the breast within 2–3 minutes of starting to pump. If this does not happen, you might try hand-expressing to trigger your let-down, and then switch to pumping when the milk starts flowing.
- When pumping, move from breast to breast as the milk stops flowing. If you massage during pumping this may help the milk to flow more efficiently. A back massage before or during expressing (using firm pressure on either side of the spine from neck to mid-back) may also assist the let-down reflex, thereby helping milk to flow. A cup of tea before expressing may also help. Tea contains a substance called theophylline which helps with oxytocin release, helping the milk to flow.

- If the breasts become overfull, pump or express more often, even every hour if necessary.
- Do not limit fluids (another old ineffective remedy often suggested to reduce milk production). Drink to thirst.

Safety measures

Bottles and equipment which will hold or have been used to feed infant formula to the baby must be sterilised thoroughly. However, breastmilk is a different product; it is not sterile, but comes with its own antibodies to specific viruses and bacteria in the mother's environment. When at home with your healthy baby, bottles which have been used to feed breastmilk need only to be washed with hot soapy water and dried with a clean tea-towel and they will be ready to use for safely feeding the next batch of breastmilk to the baby. Bottles which will be used to store frozen milk should be sterilised.

Pump parts can likewise be washed in hot soapy water 2–3 times per day, dried and used again without sterilising. It is *not* necessary to sterilise breast pumps which only the mother has used. Furthermore, it is possible to use a breast pump again without washing it at all as long as it was only used a few hours ago; simply put your used pump in a clean resealable plastic bag in your fridge and use it again without washing it, whenever you're ready to pump next time. This can save you hours of time.

Feeding expressed breastmilk

The baby will require the following quantities of breastmilk in order to grow well and thrive, as evidenced by good weight gain (see Chapter 13).

Day 1:	~30 ml colostrum (28g = 1oz)
Day 2:	60ml per kilogram per day
Day 3:	90ml per kilogram per day
Day 4:	120ml per kilogram per day
Day 5–10:	150ml per kilogram per day
From Day 10:	180ml per kilogram per day

Usually the above daily requirements are divided into 8 or 10 feeds (which may be taken at irregular intervals). For example, a baby born weighing 3kg would require the following quantities of milk:

Day 1:	~2-3 ml colostrum	8-10 times per day
Day 2:	~25ml	8 times per 24 hours
Day 3:	~35ml	8 times per 24 hours
Day 4:	~45ml	8 times per 24 hours
Day 5-10:	~55ml	8 times per 24 hours
From Day 10:	~65–70ml, or even more	approx 8 times per 24 hours

Method of feeding

Expressed breastmilk can be fed to the baby by spoon, cup,[8-11] or bottle or by supplemental nursing system, or finger-feeding.

Spoon-feeding

This is a good way to feed colostrum to a newborn. You can hand-express directly into the spoon and feed the drops to the baby straight away. For larger quantities, have the milk close to you in a cup; offer little spoonfuls with the tip of the spoon placed on the baby's lower lip and allow the baby to drink each half-spoonful.

Cup-feeding

Cup-feeding is an underutilised method of feeding newborns and pre-term babies; it may seem scary, but once you know how, it is quick and easy, and safer than bottle-feeding:

- swaddle the baby to keep his hands away from his chin
- half sit him up and place the rim of the cup on his lower lip
- tip the cup so that the milk just reaches the baby's mouth but doesn't overwhelm him
- wait for him to lap the milk
- give the baby short pauses to rest and catch his breath
- allow him to stop when he seems to tire or falls asleep.

Bottle-feeding

In order to avoid confusing the baby who is learning to breastfeed, feeding with a bottle is not generally recommended, However, whenever there is a breastfeeding difficulty which prevents the baby feeding directly at the breast, the most important thing is to feed the baby by the easiest method; 'nipple confusion' can usually be much more easily reversed once the baby is getting enough to eat (see Chapter 6):

- if expressed breastmilk has to be used for more than just a few days, mothers (and fathers if they are helping) may become impatient with other methods of feeding
- some practitioners recommend paced bottle-feeding, which allows the baby to be bottle-fed in a way believed to be more likely to preserve breastfeeding. This method slows down the flow of milk into the teat and the mouth, allowing the baby to eat more slowly, and take breaks.
  Use a slow-flow teat and pause feeding every few sucks to allow the baby to rest and so that he doesn't finish the milk very quickly
- alternatively, in order to make the transition to breastfeeding easier, other practitioners recommend making bottle-feeding as brief as possible to ensure that the baby spends the minimum amount of time becoming programmed on to the bottle. So their recommendation would be to bottle-feed the baby any supplements with a fast-flow teat, being careful that he doesn't choke and watching for signs of stress (like frowning or splayed fingers) which would tell you he needs a slower flow and frequent rests to catch his breath
- If you are planning to stop breastfeeding at six months, your baby will still have strong sucking needs and you can bear this in mind as you plan for the future. It will be easier for you, and for him, if he is already familiar with how to bottle-feed and is perhaps used to sucking on a dummy for comfort-sucking, so that changing to formula-feeding by bottle will not be too traumatic for him. It is advisable, therefore, to accustom your

baby to receive an occasional feed of breastmilk by bottle, perhaps 2–3 times a week and starting before he has become too opinionated about receiving all of his milk at the breast.

Supplemental nursing system

Babies can be tube-fed expressed milk at the breast via a thin tube taped beside the nipple attached to a feeding bottle. This allows him to receive extra milk at the breast. The supplementer container holds the milk, which travels through a tube into your baby's mouth while he breastfeeds. As he swallows, he continues suckling, stimulating your milk production.[13]

Finger-feeding

When the baby needs to receive expressed milk, parents often develop a team approach with the mother pumping and the father doing the finger-feeding, which can work really well until the baby is able to breastfeed direct.

- The baby sucks on the mother's (or father's) finger, pad side up.
- Have the milk in a cup.
- The milk is offered beside the finger through a syringe, a dropper, or supplemental nursing tube inserted into the corner of the baby's mouth.[14]
- If using a syringe or dropper, it can be removed from the baby's mouth with the other hand, dipped into the cup, refilled and re-inserted into the baby's mouth without removing the finger that the baby is sucking.

11: PASTEURISATION/FLASH-HEATING BREASTMILK

When there are valid concerns about unsafe levels of HIV in breastmilk, or infections suffered by mother or baby that could pose a risk factor for transmission of the virus to the breastfed baby, the suggestion is frequently made by cautious physicians that mothers with HIV should stop breastfeeding and switch the baby to formula. The British HIV Association says,

> *If HIV virus becomes detectable in your blood: stop breast/chestfeeding and start using formula milk. Do not use milk you have expressed and stored. Feed your baby using formula only. Your baby may need to take anti-HIV medication as post exposure prophylaxis. Contact your clinic team to discuss this urgently. If your baby is unwell with diarrhoea and/ or vomiting: feed your baby with formula milk only while your baby is unwell. As it can be difficult to know when the baby's gut lining has fully recovered, we do not advise restarting breast/chestfeeding, but continuing formula milk. Contact your HIV team for advice on what to do.[1]*
>
> *…If you have diarrhoea or vomiting, or a breast/chest injury or infection: stop breast/chestfeeding and feed your baby with formula milk OR use milk that you expressed more than 2 days (48 hours) before your tummy or breast problem began…*

However, if the baby is found to need formula supplements for any reason, concerns about the risk of HIV-transmission due to mixed breast and bottle-feeding make the use of partial formula-feeding unsafe, causing worries that the mother may need to switch over to complete formula-feeding.

Weaning from the breast is not always necessary. Heat-treated or home-pasteurised mother's own milk is a logical and feasible way to continue safely providing your baby with breastmilk, usually on a temporary basis, until you can return to exclusive breastfeeding at the breast. Heat-treatment of breastmilk using simple equipment is not only safe, but possible.

The benefits to the baby of heat-treated breastmilk vs formula

Heat-treated expressed breastmilk (EBM) has many advantages over formula (as outlined in Chapter 4). Breastmilk is:

- Physiologically normal for the human baby
- Immunologically protective
- Nutritionally perfect (some components are slightly changed)
- Non-allergenic
- Free from harmful bacteria and viruses
- Free
- Feasible
- Compatible with current WHO infant feeding guidance since it enables exclusive breastmilk-feeding for six months.

Pasteurising breastmilk at home

Home pasteurisation using simple equipment available in any kitchen is safe and possible. It is the most logical feeding alternative for those women who wish to avoid any possibility of transmission of HIV to their babies through breastfeeding, yet wish to provide them with the most suitable milk. Mother's milk is tailor-made and no replacement or substitute infant milks can come close to the unique nutritional benefits that mothers bestow on their babies during breastfeeding.

The mother who provides her own milk for her baby also has absolute control over her own milk supply and can assure her baby's food security in uncertain times. Heat-treated EBM is nutritionally superior to other replacement feeds, maintains some immunological protection, avoids the risk of allergy, and is always available.

Research confirming the safety of pasteurised breastmilk

Banked human milk is made safe by a method called Holder pasteurisation, whereby the milk is heated to a temperature of 62.5

degrees C in a water-bath for 30 minutes. In a 1993 study done for the Human Milk Banking Association of North America researchers found that HIV could be inactivated by Holder pasteurisation.[2] The first study to find that home pasteurisation of breastmilk would also inactivate HIV was conducted in Puerto Rico by Dr Caroline Chantry in 2000.[3] Although HIV could be identified in the milk of 88% of the women, it could not be recovered from any of the samples after a method of pasteurisation which they called flash-boiling (see below for method). A South African researcher called Bridget Jeffery also looked at a similar method of home-pasteurisation called Pretoria pasteurisation to inactivate HIV in 2000 and 2001.[4,5,6] Studies published in 2005 and 2008 comparing the safety of flash-heating and Pretoria pasteurisation found that flash-heating was somewhat more efficient, destroyed *E. coli* or *S. aureus* contamination, and conserved more of the milk's components.[7,8]

Further studies

Further studies confirmed that flash-heating, a simple method of heating milk in a pan of water on a stove, can inactivate HIV in naturally infected breastmilk,[9,10] and that nutritional components were not significantly affected.[11,12] Flash-heating was effective against bacterial contamination and afterwards the milk could be stored at room temperature for 6–8 hours.[13,14] It was concluded that most breastmilk immunoglobulin activity survives flash-heating, suggesting that it is immunologically superior to breastmilk substitutes.[15]

Overseas use of flash-heated breastmilk

The use of pasteurised expressed breastmilk was officially endorsed by the Zimbabwe Ministry of Health as a primary option to be considered by HIV+ mothers.[16] Hospitals in Pretoria and Durban,[17] South Africa, have used pasteurised breastmilk to feed newborns. In Tanzania flash-heating has been used after exclusive breastfeeding, while avoiding HIV transmission associated with non-exclusive breastfeeding.[18] The ZVITAMBO project in rural

Zimbabwe[19] ascertained the feasibility of expressing and heat-treating all breastmilk fed to HIV-exposed, uninfected infants following six months of exclusive breastfeeding. Flash-heating may be of particular value during times of greater risk for mother-to-child-transmission, such as during episodes of infant oral thrush, maternal mastitis, or interrupted antiretroviral prophylaxis and/or during the addition of complementary foods.[20]

Using heat-treated expressed breastmilk as an emergency feeding method

Mothers can use flash-heated breastmilk to feed the baby in the following scenarios:

- For exclusive breastmilk-feeding (from birth, instead of breastfeeding directly if there are concerns about viral levels in breastmilk)
- As a temporary measure, where there is concern that direct breastfeeding may infect the baby,[21] e.g.
  > In the case of maternal viral blips, when there are concerns that the mother's ART is not effective, or if for some reason she has not been adherent
  > If the mother is suffering from mastitis, or has sore nipples
- To avoid mixed feeding if babies are not gaining enough weight and might need supplemental formula top-ups
- To assist healing and avoid the risk of transmission of HIV when the baby's gut may have been damaged by
  > a gastrointestinal infection, diarrhoea
  > allergy or sensitivity causing intestinal bleeding
- For a baby who has had a frenotomy or oral thrush with bleeding in the mouth
- To avoid the risk of mixed feeding if the baby has received solid foods too early (before six months)
- During the changeover period when a mother intends to prematurely wean her baby from the breast and on to other foods/liquids/formula. In order to avoid effectively mixing

breast and formula-feeding, the mother living with HIV should consider the possibility of feeding her pasteurised breastmilk for several days before commencing exclusive formula-feeding
- For informally donated breastmilk to ensure safety for the recipient baby
- To provide a safe change-over from bottle to breast when there has been a decision to reverse previous formula-feeding, e.g.
  > if hospital staff have started bottle-feeding a newborn without the mother's permission and she wishes to breastfeed
  > if the mother herself has decided to opt for breastfeeding after a short period of formula-feeding

Note: In these situations, if it's possible that a baby's gut has already been damaged by previous formula-feeding, it's necessary to allow time for it to heal. Maureen Minchin, international expert in infant gut health and author of *Milk Matters: Infant Feeding and Immune Disorder*,[22] has expressed the opinion that healing can take three weeks. Thus it is suggested that this is the length of time that the baby would need to receive heat-treated expressed breastmilk *after all formula feeding is over*, and before breastfeeding direct is initiated or resumed.
- HIV clinicians and paediatricians are often reassured to know that this safe alternative exists and can be used if something unexpected happens during the course of breastfeeding.

Pasteurising breastmilk

Method 1: Flash-heating
- Place 50–120ml milk in a clean covered 455ml glass jar.
- Place the jar upright in a small pan of cold water. The level of water in the pan should be two finger-widths above the level of the milk in the jar. Importantly, the amount of milk should not exceed 120ml – research has not verified safety above this amount.
- Place the pan on the stove and heat until the water reaches a rolling boil. In order to ensure it reaches a high enough temperature, ensure that the water boils for 1½ to 2 minutes

before the pan is removed from the heat.
- Remove the pan from the heat and remove the jar from the hot water.[23]
- Cover the milk with the lid of the jar.
- Cool rapidly by placing in a bowl of cold water with ice added and then feed to the baby when it is cool. (Rapid cooling prevents further breakdown of immune properties.)

Method 2: Pretoria pasteurisation
- Place 50ml–150ml milk into a clean glass jar and cover.
- Boil 450ml water in a small pot, and remove from the heat-source.
- Place the covered milk jar upright in the pan of boiled water, cover the pan and leave for 15–20 minutes before removing. The milk may be fed to the baby once cooled.

Note about pasteurisation of colostrum:
This aspect of pasteurisation has not yet been researched. Very small quantities of milk, such as colostrum, may dry/congeal in the container during pasteurisation. It may be necessary to add 5–10ml (1–2 teaspoons) of cooled boiled water to the pasteurised colostrum before feeding it by teaspoon in tiny quantities (drop by drop) to the baby. As soon as the quantity of colostrum increases so that it remains liquid in the container, it is preferable to stop adding extra water. Breastmilk production increases dramatically within the first 36–72 hours after birth, and exclusive pasteurised-breastmilk-feeding (i.e. no other foods, no other liquids) is best for the baby for the first six months of life.

Storing pasteurised breastmilk
- Raw, unpasteurised expressed breastmilk should be stored in covered containers as shown in Chapter 10.
- Breastmilk which has been pasteurised will not keep as long as raw milk. It may be safely stored in the fridge, or in a covered jar at room temperature (~23°C) for eight hours afterwards if the jar remains unopened (i.e. so long as the milk is not subsequently

exposed to bacteria from hands or other containers).[12]
- If frozen and thawed, ensure the milk is used within 48 hours.[24]

SECTION III

TROUBLESHOOTING

12. BREAST PROBLEMS

Breast problems, in particular those related to over-supply of breastmilk, such as engorgement, some types of sore nipples, mastitis and abscess, are not always inevitable and – if a mother is able to 'manage' her own breastmilk supply carefully as described in Chapter 7 – they should be entirely preventable. However, in spite of the best plans, sometimes things can go wrong and mothers who live with HIV need special care because of the risk of transmission of the virus to their infants during breastfeeding. In particular:

- breast engorgement may increase breast permeability leading to elevated viral levels in breastmilk
- before routine treatment with antiretroviral therapy, breast or nipple problems were estimated to double the risk of transmission of HIV to the breastfed baby[1]
- a compromised immune system increases the risk of mastitis
- unrelieved engorgement may reduce breastmilk storage capacity, compromising a mother's ability to exclusively breastfeed for a full six months

Breast care if the baby is not breastfeeding

If the baby is not breastfeeding well (or at all), then it's important that the mother express or pump both breasts at least as often as a newborn would want to feed (every three hours, or even more often). See Chapter 10 for how to express and pump:

- to produce milk to feed the baby by another method (e.g. cup, spoon, bottle as described in Chapter 14)
- to drain the breasts

Causes of engorgement

The breasts can become overfull any time more milk is being made than is being drained. Common causes are:

- over-production of milk during Lactogenesis II, especially days 4–9 after birth
- a sleepy, sick, jaundiced or premature baby who is not breastfeeding effectively
- sore nipples (the mother shortens or delays breastfeeds because of the pain)
- mastitis or abscess (cause or consequence)
- mother-baby separation (for work or social events)
- baby sleeping longer times (naps or at night)
- change in family routine (holidays, visiting relatives)
- older baby becoming easily distracted
- nursing strike (sudden breast refusal by the baby)
- sleep-training programmes, leaving baby to cry it out (not recommended!)
- fast weaning
- pumping frequency changes for those mothers not breastfeeding direct or attempting to create a freezer-stash of expressed breastmilk (e.g. pump a lot one day and a lot less the next)

Consequences of engorgement

Overproduction of breastmilk is called engorgement when the breasts become hot, heavy and uncomfortable. It is one of the most common breastfeeding problems in the early postpartum. If no intervention is made, continued breastmilk production will make the breasts hard, wooden, shiny and even inflamed. The mother herself may become feverish as the situation becomes more and more urgent. Thereafter over-production of breastmilk – if ignored – can lead to a cascade of further problems, as shown:

BREASTFEEDING POSITIVELY

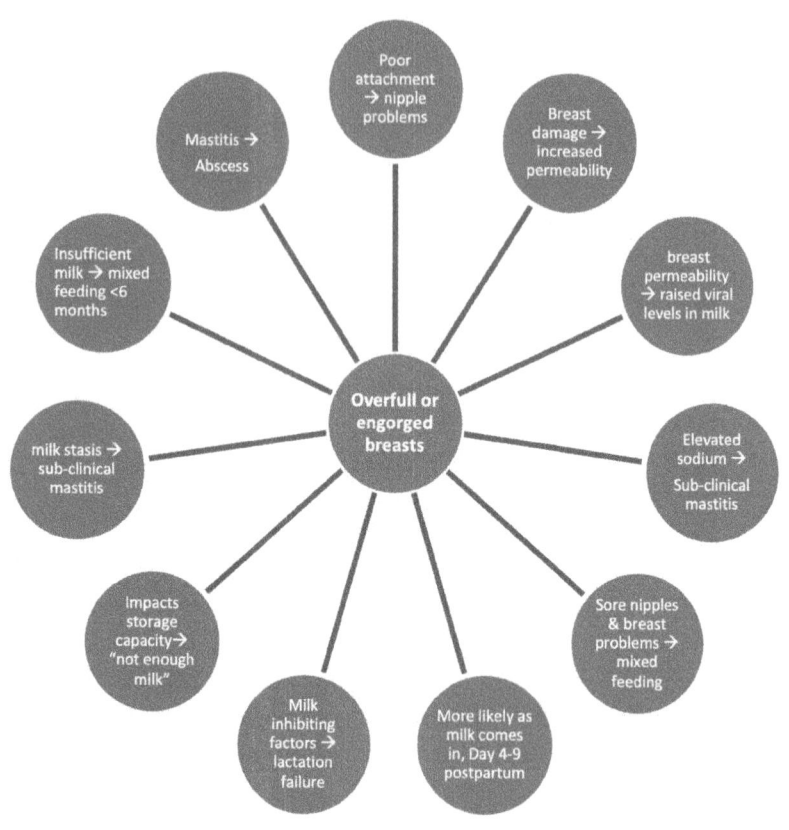

Central node: **Overfull or engorged breasts**, connected to:
- Poor attachment → nipple problems
- Breast damage → increased permeability
- breast permeability → raised viral levels in milk
- Elevated sodium → Sub-clinical mastitis
- Sore nipples & breast problems → mixed feeding
- More likely as milk comes in, Day 4-9 postpartum
- Milk inhibiting factors → lactation failure
- Impacts storage capacity → "not enough milk"
- milk stasis → sub-clinical mastitis
- Insufficient milk → mixed feeding <6 months
- Mastitis → Abscess

Source: Morrison P, developed for WABA HIV Kit 2018.

Conflicting information about over-production of milk

Unfortunately, the mother who is starting to experience overfull breasts is often told that if she attempts to relieve the pressure by expressing or pumping, then she will go on producing too much milk. In the past, out-of-date advice included recommendations to bind the breasts, limit fluids and take paracetamol. Today, friends or relations may suggest that a mother just put up with the pain and discomfort and on no account drain her breasts, for her own good. While it may be well-meaning, this is poor advice because:

- milk goes on being produced for several days before a small protein in the milk (called feedback inhibitor of lactation, or FIL)

sends a clear message to the milk-producing cells to make less, so over-fullness becomes engorgement, and mild engorgement becomes severe
- the fuller the breasts the more difficult it is to drain them; the pressure within the cells prevents oxytocin, the hormone that causes the milk-ejection reflex, from acting on the little basket-like cells surrounding the lactocytes (milk-producing cells) to expel the milk into the ducts and down towards the nipple, where it can be expressed
- the milk-producing cells may become over-distended, press against each other and burst, causing severe damage and pain
- tight junctions between the cells and the blood vessels may open, allowing mixing of blood plasma and milk, with a risk of elevated HIV viral levels in the milk
- with little or no nipple stimulation, prolactin levels plummet, which, with the increasing risk of inflammation, cause the mother to become depressed (physiologically this is similar to what would happen if the baby died)
- milk stasis (when the milk remains in the breast) encourages proliferation of pathogenic bacteria and leads to an increased risk for mastitis, which in turn can be a risk factor for breast abscess
- eventually, unresolved engorgement leads to severely compromised breastmilk production as the milk-producing cells shut down, ultimately leading to the need for the baby to receive supplemental feeding.[2] For a mother living with HIV this would require immediate weaning since mixed feeding before six months is a risk factor for mother-to-child transmission
- long-term engorgement for 10 days–2 weeks leads to lactation failure; the breasts feel much softer as they stop producing milk, and the undrained milk is reabsorbed.

The reasons for resolving engorgement:
- maintain breast integrity and prevent damage to the milk-producing cells

- prevent elevated viral levels in the milk
- soften the breast and areola to ensure that it is graspable by the baby, i.e. he can continue to latch and breastfeed
- enable the baby to be fed expressed breastmilk for the time that latching is difficult or impossible

How to resolve engorgement

It cannot be over-emphasised that most breast engorgement is completely avoidable. The best preventive measure is to breastfeed often from birth. If the baby is too sleepy or too full, then the mother will have to drain the breasts herself. Over-fullness or engorgement is very easy to prevent or resolve, but the urgency of the situation needs to be recognised. Act quickly; don't leave it! It helps if you have already arranged for the use of a good-quality breast pump – see Chapter 3)

- Wake the baby to breastfeed whenever the breasts feel even just a *little* too full, even if this is very often.
- *During* breastfeeding, whenever the baby takes a pause, use *breast compression* to drain the breasts and increase the baby's intake:
    > using the hand supporting the breast, give a gentle squeeze or a very slight lift of the breast to trigger another let-down of milk and another sucking burst
    > allow the baby to drink for as long as he will without squeezing the breast
    > when the baby takes another pause, gently squeeze the breast again
    > If the baby has gone to sleep, you can tickle behind his ears with your finger and thumb when using the cross-cradle hold, or blow on his face if you don't have a spare hand available to stimulate him
    > don't tickle his cheek or stimulate his face, as this can cause him to unlatch and turn towards the stimulus and away from the breast

- *After* breastfeeding, if the breasts still seem uncomfortable or overfull, then express or pump whatever milk the baby leaves behind, no matter how much that is (store it in the fridge, not in the breasts)
- In the first few days after birth, some of the breast over-fullness may be oedema; it can be helpful if, after breastfeeding or expressing or pumping, you are able to lie flat on your back with your arms above your head, to help allow drainage of some of the extra fluid from your breasts
- If the baby is too sleepy to breastfeed frequently to drain your breasts, start expressing or pumping instead (save the milk in case he wakes up hungry!)

Gentle breast massage can assist drainage
- *gently* massage the whole breast, area by area,
- massage from the back near the ribs, and from as far up as your armpit towards the nipple
- use little finger-tip circles, *or* gentle pressure with your knuckles
- lean forward to reach and massage any firm areas underneath the breast
- If there are any hard lumpy areas remaining, massage them gently, and express/pump again

Alternate massage and pumping and keep going until the whole breast is soft and comfortable. How soft? The areola should feel as soft as your earlobe, not as hard as the tip of your nose.

- The breasts will 'fill' again very soon. There is nothing you can do to prevent this; you can only help resolve it by expressing or pumping as often as it takes, every hour if necessary.
- Warmth (warm wet flannels, a warm bath/shower) before pumping can help milk to 'flow'.
- Cold (ice-packs) or cabbage leaves applied around the breasts after pumping can reduce swelling (oedema), helping to suppress lactation and reduce inflammation. As described in

Chapter 7, use an ordinary white round cabbage; wash and dry the leaves and keep them in a clean plastic bag in the fridge. Tuck the leaves/cold-packs inside the bra or T-shirt. Change the leaves every couple of hours or when they go limp. Stop using the cabbage when your breasts are comfortable.
- Parsley or sage are herbal remedies used in salads or stuffings as a natural lactation suppressant.
- If wished, wear a loose bra or close-fitting T-shirt to provide support to full breasts. However, do not apply extra pressure by wearing a too-tight bra, or by 'binding' the breasts (this information is outdated and harmful, as explained above).

Storing and feeding expressed breastmilk from an engorged breast

If the engorgement has not lasted very long:

- Any extra expressed milk can be stored in the fridge or frozen; don't throw it away.
- Stored expressed breastmilk can be fed to the baby, but if he will breastfeed direct that is preferable.
- If the baby is not breastfeeding at all, he should receive expressed milk by cup, spoon or bottle (quantities are given in Chapter 10).
- If the breast has been engorged for some time, and due to the risk of transmission of HIV from elevated viral levels in the milk, it may be necessary to pasteurise any expressed milk before feeding it to the baby. More information on pasteurising and feeding expressed milk to the baby can be found in Chapters 10 and 11.

Blocked ducts

If a particular area of the breast is not draining well it may block the area behind it and prevent it from draining. So we call this a 'blocked duct'. It feels like a firm area which seems to stay uncomfortably full, and it may also be tender or painful. To help resolve it:

- Breastfeed the baby from the affected breast as often as you can
- Have the baby's chin pointing towards the blockage, if possible,

since the tongue is most effective at draining the affected area
- Gently massage the affected breast, over and behind the lumpy area, and express, massage and express again, until it becomes soft
- You can try massaging the breast in a basin of warm water, or in a warm bath, which helps the milk to 'flow'
- Express as much milk as you can from that breast to keep it as empty as possible
- In between expressing sessions, place a piece of cool, clean cabbage leaf inside your bra, over the blocked duct (not over the whole breast) – this may help to suppress lactation in that area
- Don't ignore a blocked duct, since it can progress to mastitis. So do all that you can to clear it as soon as possible.[3]
- After the problem has resolved, treat the affected breast respectfully in the next few days – maybe feed from that side first and if necessary express after feeding. Don't allow it to become overfull.

How breast pathology increases
risk of HIV through breastfeeding

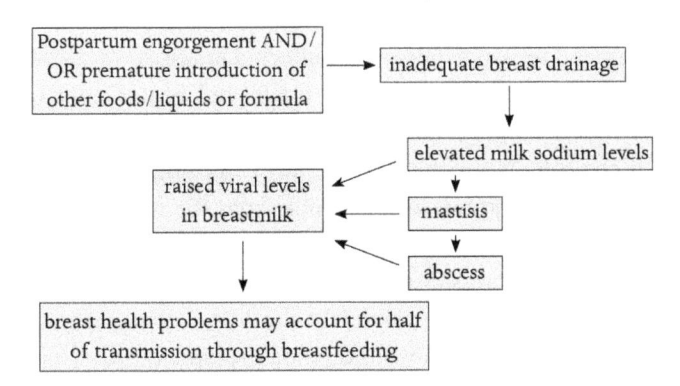

Postpartum engorgement AND/OR premature introduction of other foods/liquids or formula → inadequate breast drainage → elevated milk sodium levels → mastisis → abscess → raised viral levels in breastmilk → breast health problems may account for half of transmission through breastfeeding

Mastitis and sub-clinical mastitis

Outside the context of HIV, mastitis is fairly common, and it often follows having allowed a sore or lumpy area of the breast to remain undrained. Mastitis is:

- experienced by almost one-third of breastfeeding mothers,[4,5]
- usually occurs in only one breast
- is most often experienced in the first seven weeks after birth, starting within 2–3 weeks,[2] related to poor breastfeeding practices leading to breast engorgement and milk stasis
- infective or non-infective
- associated with raised HIV levels in breastmilk and risk of transmission to the baby.[6-8]

Symptoms of mastitis

- a firm lumpy area within the breast (induration) as opposed to a normal cobblestone texture
- pain
- inflammation (may be faint; it's easier to see if you look in a mirror)
- fever (temperature > 38°C)
- malaise, e.g. you feel really sick and weepy.

What to do to help resolve mastitis

- rest! Go to bed and take the baby with you. Arrange for someone else to take over all your responsibilities except for baby-care.
- suspend breastfeeding on the affected breast
- breastfeed the baby on the unaffected breast only until all symptoms have resolved and for several days afterwards
- if the baby is still hungry after breastfeeding, feed the baby on pasteurised expressed breastmilk from the affected breast (see Chapters 11 and 13)
- alternate expressing/pumping with gentle massage of the affected breast to completely drain it; keep going until the whole breast is as soft and drained as possible
  > every two hours while you are awake
  > every three hours at night
- use massage before pumping and cabbage afterwards (as described above for a blocked duct)
- if the breast is not a lot better within 24 hours and if pain and

fever are not resolved, seek medical advice *the same day*. Ask the doctor about the advisability of a course of antibiotics to treat the mastitis. Do not leave it! If necessary go to A & E at your local hospital
- during mastitis, milk samples can be analysed for a bacterial infection. Sometimes the doctor will take a milk sample first and send it for testing but prescribe an antibiotic the same day anyway, and check if it is appropriate against the results when they come back from the lab. The lab report will identify the bacteria, and indicate antibiotic sensitivity or resistance to the infection, so the doctor knows whether you should continue with the medication already prescribed, or whether it needs to be changed. This reduces any delay in treating a breast infection, saving pain and discomfort as well as limiting the amount of time that direct breastfeeding might need to be temporarily suspended
- even if you are prescribed an antibiotic, it's important that you *continue to keep the breast as well drained as you can until all symptoms have resolved* (i.e. the pain is gone and the lumpy area is soft)
- expect symptoms to resolve in reverse order
  > fever and malaise
  > inflammation
  > pain/discomfort
  > induration (a lumpy area)
- you may find that during mastitis the quantity of breastmilk you produce seems quite a lot less due to the affected area being unable to drain. Keeping the rest of the breast very well drained for several days will have the effect of increasing breastmilk production. Mothers are often concerned that this will cause over-production. However, once the mastitis is completely resolved, too much milk can be addressed by allowing the breast to stay just a little too full. See more about suppressing lactation in Chapter 14.

Abscess

Breast abscess doesn't just happen; it is a progression:

> Over-fullness → engorgement → mastitis → abscess

Having an abscess is the worst breast problem that you can experience during breastfeeding. It eventually becomes a medical emergency requiring close medical supervision. There is often a need for multiple courses of antibiotics followed by surgery, leaving a painful and messy open wound which leaks milk for weeks. Alternatively, if the abscess is small it may be treated by needle aspiration, which may need to be repeated several times. In the context of HIV you would already have had to stop breastfeeding from the affected breast due to previous mastitis. A mother living with HIV who wanted to work through the aftercare to resume breastfeeding later would need to maintain meticulous drainage of the breast, and probably discard the milk until the infection is over.

In fact, abscess should be completely preventable; the key is breast drainage. Do all that you can to avoid an abscess, and seek medical treatment way before it comes to that.

Unexplained breast pain

Breast pain without other symptoms is unusual, but it can happen. The nerves from the back radiate around to the breast, and unexplained breast pain needs to be investigated by a doctor.

13. NIPPLE PROBLEMS

Special care if you have HIV

The most common reason for a breastfeeding mother to start supplementing with formula, or to abandon breastfeeding altogether, is pain during breastfeeding. There can be several causes of sore nipples[1] and some of them are quite rare. But there are many strategies and techniques that a mother can use to avoid the inevitability of this painful condition.

Mothers living with HIV need to be especially careful to avoid or resolve sore or bleeding nipples because:

- contact between the mother's blood and the baby's mouth is a risk factor for transmission of the virus,[2,3] and there is more about this in Chapter 2.
- sore nipples can provide an entry point for bacterial infection of the breast, i.e. mastitis, which in itself is another risk factor for HIV transmission to the breastfed baby.[4]
- supplementing with formula means practising mixed feeding, which has been found to double the risk of HIV transmission.[5]

Your comfort

At the first hint of pain, review all your positioning and latching techniques and be prepared to change something so that breastfeeding is more comfortable. Importantly, if you have HIV and want to continue breastfeeding, rather than switching to the bottle, these problems cannot be left to get worse. They need to be addressed very quickly.

Your comfort is important. The most common reason for pain is that the baby is positioned poorly at the breast. The nipple shape and site of any damage can reveal a lot about what may be happening inside the baby's mouth and it may be worthwhile seeking the help of an IBCLC to identify the cause.

Pain can be used to identify what could be going wrong. When the baby is latched, how does it feel? The first suck or two may feel stretchy and strong, but in fact the nipple can stretch to twice its length inside the baby's mouth, and once this happens, the tip of the nipple should reach the back of the baby's throat where it can't become damaged. If you are still feeling pain once the baby is drinking well, it's important to adjust something. You can try positioning the baby a little differently – lift him up or down, or support the breast more effectively from underneath so that he doesn't have to hang on to a heavy breast in order to breastfeed. If that doesn't work, take him off the breast and latch him again, more carefully.

Varying breastfeeding positions

If the nipples are becoming tender, it can be helpful to vary breastfeeding positions, so that the area of stress is changed. If you usually use the cradle hold, breastfeed every other feed in the football hold and vice versa.

Positioning so that you have most control

It's difficult to control where the baby's mouth is going on latching when you hold him in the cradle hold. You will have much more control if you position him in the cross-cradle or the rugby hold (see Chapter 6).

Stretching

Can you see the breast stretching in and out with each suck? Sometimes you can see the skin being stretched above the areola, or on one side or the other. This shows that the baby's mouth is poorly placed on the nipple/areola; he is not quite straight, or too high, or too low. He should take in to his mouth more of the underside of the areola than the top, but he shouldn't be so low that the nipple can't extend to the back of his palate. Sometimes you can see 'jarring' when this happens, as the baby's upper gum grazes the face of the nipple each time he closes his jaws.

To resolve this kind of positioning problem, without unlatching the baby, move him very slightly *towards* the stretching, so that it no longer happens. For instance, to resolve any 'jarring' you would need to lift him a tiny bit higher. To visualise what needs to change, imagine that the nipple is the stem of a flower and your baby's lips are the petals – are they straight, or is the stem being bent, up or down, or to one side or the other? Sometimes an observer may find this easier to see than you can – ask your partner to look and see and, without unlatching the baby, move him to straighten things out.

Negative pressure

During the first 2–3 days after birth, the breasts produce low quantities of colostrum (the first milk). This is an advantage to the baby, who doesn't need large quantities of milk at this time, and can learn to coordinate sucking, swallowing and breathing on a breast that is not producing overwhelming quantities of milk.

However, one of the things that can happen before the milk comes in is that negative pressure from the baby's sucking can cause breakdown of the nipple tissue. A baby who is hungry has a stronger suck on the nipple than one who is not hungry, so this means that the prime time for sore nipples to occur is within the first 2–3 days, while he is learning to breastfeed and before the milk comes in.[6] If he has a shallow latch, so that he is not positioned with the nipple far back in his mouth, milk transfer is compromised, so he may obtain even less colostrum than he could if he was latched well. The likelihood of sore nipples lessens as the breasts begin producing more milk. Mothers can take steps to minimise tissue damage by paying close attention to where the baby is sucking. Once the milk starts flowing, there will also be less negative pressure exerted on the nipple.

As a consequence of breast over-fullness

After the milk comes in, and especially if the baby hasn't been breastfeeding effectively, the breasts may become full and hard, which can make latching difficult or sometimes even impossible. The areola may become so hard that the nipple may become flattened and obliterated. From the baby's perspective it's like trying to attach to a balloon. A baby with a weaker suck, even if he was breastfeeding well beforehand, may now be unable to attach at all. A baby with a strong suck may latch but be unable to take a large mouthful because the tissue is too firm. Negative pressure from the strong suck may damage the face of the nipple, causing blood blisters or actual bleeding.

How full is too full? The areola should be soft and 'graspable', and as soft as your earlobe. If it is as firm as the tip of your nose, the breast is too full. The best strategy to address this is to hand express enough milk that the whole breast is soft and comfortable, with no remaining lumpy areas, and the areola softens so that the nipple becomes graspable once again. In the meantime, feed your expressed breastmilk to the baby in another way (see Chapter 14). Keep on expressing and feeding expressed milk for as long as it takes to keep the breasts soft and the milk flowing well. (See more on how to manage engorgement in Chapter 12).

A short latch

The most likely cause of sore nipples is that the baby is taking a short latch. A baby who is latched well should take an asymmetric mouthful of breast tissue (more of the underneath in than the top). So his chin should be dug well into the breast below the areola and his nose should be just touching on top. When he is well latched, the first couple of sucks might feel quite strong as he stretches the nipple to the back of his throat, but then it should feel comfortable and the mother should feel no pain. If breastfeeding is painful, something about the latch will need to be changed.

Re-latching

Sometimes mothers who know about the importance of latching so that breastfeeding is comfortable attempt to latch and re-latch many times, trying to encourage the baby to take a larger mouthful of breast tissue. This often works well. However, if you take him off the breast too often, the baby will become very frustrated, then his tongue lifts as he cries, and he becomes more and more difficult to latch. Babies learn very quickly and sometimes they learn to expect trouble, so working to make breastfeeding as easy for the baby as possible can be very worthwhile.

If your baby becomes upset about being taken off the breast too often, calm him down before you try again, and improve his latch by adjusting his position in relation to the breast *after* he is already on the breast. Lift the breast very slightly, or drop the breast lower, or bring the baby closer to your armpit, or tuck his body closer to your tummy and see if it improves your comfort first without upsetting him.

Wetting the nipple/areola and the baby's mouth

A relatively easy way to help a good latch, especially if your baby seems to slurp on to the breast and you have difficulty in encouraging him to take a wide gape before you bring him on to the breast is to:

- express a drop or two of milk before you start latching (see Chapter 10 on expressing)
- use the drops to wet the nipple and areola, *and* the baby's lips, so that everything is slippery
- when he takes his first big suck on latching, the nipple can then slide easily into the back of the baby's throat where it can't become damaged
- once latched, his chin should be dug well in with his nose just touching the breast on top
- you will need to support the breast well.

Supporting the breast throughout the feed

Once the baby is latched, try supporting the breast as if you are 'pouring' it into his mouth from the back near your ribs. This has the effect of flattening the underside of the breast so that he can take more of the underneath in. While there is any nipple tenderness, you should support the breast thoughout the entire feed.

Clicking

If the baby makes a clicking sound with each suck it indicates that he is losing suction; the weight of the heavy breast can drag on the baby's lower jaw and he loses the breast (and has to slurp it back in again causing friction). To remedy this, the baby needs to be encouraged to take a deeper latch with a wide gape as he goes on to the breast, and you should support the breast well.

Positional sore stripe and lipstick-shaped nipple

How does the nipple look immediately the baby unlatches? Is it shaped like a lipstick, with a flattened area on the underside of the nipple tapering to a wedge at the tip (a positional sore stripe)? If so, the baby is latched too high, and he needs to take more of the underside of the nipple and areola into his mouth. It's also likely that the breast is not being supported effectively. You need to cup the breast underneath to take the weight of the heavy breast off the baby's lower jaw, so that the nipple doesn't come forward in the baby's mouth, enabling him to keep a larger mouthful of breast tissue deep in his mouth.

Nipple abrasions

A short latch can cause the whole face of the nipple to become abraded. Sometimes a very tiny area of abrasion can become visible right in the centre of the nipple and it may bleed. Once again, ensuring the baby takes a larger mouthful of breast tissue, and supporting the breast well throughout the feed, will resolve the problem.

Cracks where the nipple meets the areola

These extremely painful cracks can be caused by too much stretching and over time the skin splits open. If there is bleeding, you will need to express the milk from that breast and 'rest' that nipple until it heals (see Chapter 10 on feeding EBM). Healing is slow because the cracks may split with each breastfeed and seem to heal from the base of the 'V' instead of healing closed, as you would like. When you resume breastfeeding, something about the way you position your baby at the breast will also need to change to avoid the problem happening again. Check that your baby is straight on to the breast. Is there any stretching that you can see? If so, move the baby or the breast so that it stops.

Another way to track down the cause of cracked nipples is to imagine that the areola is a clock…

- if the crack is happening on the right breast from 9 to 11 o'clock then you're probably holding the baby too far over towards your left breast; move him closer to your armpit so that the stretching stops.
- If the crack is underneath, say where your baby's tongue is placed from 4 to 6 o'clock (this is the most painful condition), then the baby may be positioned too high. Try lifting the breast slightly, in line with the baby's smile. Check too that the baby is held tummy to tummy with you and that his body is close and that his hands are away from his chest.

When there are cracks on the side of the nipple, it's possible to reduce the stress on a particular area and hasten healing by positioning the baby so that the *corner* of his mouth is closest to the site of the crack. So if you usually use the cradle hold, change to the rugby hold for a few days, or vice versa.

Bacterial infection

One of the least mentioned causes of nipple pain in the popular literature is the possibility of a bacterial infection. Yet a bacterial infection can cause ongoing, exquisite pain. The mother might have either:

- nipple abrasions or cracks which go on and on; despite adjusting her positioning and being careful about how she latches the baby, the nipple simply doesn't heal
- alternatively, there can be no visible damage at all except that

the nipple looks slightly more pink than usual, but there is exquisite pain.

Here is where you need urgent extra help and medical advice:

- consult an experienced breastfeeding counsellor or IBCLC for more help to rule out a positioning problem; ensure that they know that you are breastfeeding with HIV because continued breastfeeding during severe nipple damage (as is sometimes encouraged outside the context of HIV) would not be appropriate for you
- consider asking your doctor to take a nipple swab, or a milk sample, to be sent to the lab for bacterial analysis. The lab may be able to identify a staphylococcal or a streptococcal infection, as well as providing your doctor with a list of antibiotics which are resistant or sensitive to the particular organism. Sometimes a second or even a third course of oral antibiotics may be necessary if the pain doesn't resolve with one course
- topical antibiotic ointments or creams are often prescribed, but don't seem to be very effective
- If there is any reluctance to complete these tests, or issue repeat prescriptions, it is advisable to contact your multidisciplinary team for more help, or seek a second opinion from another doctor
- It should not be necessary to wean; an alternative is to rest this nipple, express your milk, pasteurise it and feed it by another method until the nipple heals and/or the pain resolves (see Chapter 14).

Thrush

Nipple cracks are especially likely if you have a thrush infection of the nipples. Also known as *Candida albicans*, thrush can be extremely painful.

- The skin on the nipple or areola can look red, angry, shiny, and

it can tear easily.
- The baby may also have white patches on his tongue or inside his lips.
- Thrush can be confused with a bacterial infection, and so a doctor should make the diagnosis and will usually prescribe medication for the mother and for the baby.
- Both mother and baby need to be treated to avoid passing the infection back and forth between you.
- Thrush is very contagious. You will need to wash your hands after handling your breasts, change bra pads frequently, launder bras often and hang them in the sun to dry, and use clean towels every day.

Tongue and other ties

Oral ties are often blamed for breastfeeding difficulties, especially a latching difficulty, sore nipples or low weight gain.[7]

- Tongue-tie, also known by the Latin name *ankyloglossia*, describes a shorter-than-normal membrane (the frenulum) which anchors the baby's tongue to the floor of his mouth.[8] The tongue may look heart-shaped when he cries
- 'Posterior tongue-tie' is believed to anchor the back third of the tongue
- 'Labial frenulum' is a tie connecting the upper gum to the upper lip, or the lower gum to the lower lip)
- 'Buccal ties' are ties connecting the cheeks to the gums

There is concern that ties may cause speech impediments or affect dental hygiene later because the tongue can't reach to the roof of the mouth or move freely from side to side. Recommendations include surgical or laser division of the tie, known as frenotomy. However, opinion is very divided about how often ankyloglossia actually occurs, and how much it impacts successful and comfortable latching and breastfeeding.[9,10]

David Elad, writing on tongue-tie, observed that the baby's

tongue only needs to lift 3–4mm from the floor of the mouth during active breastfeeding.[11] He wrote, *'The anterior tongue, which is wedged between the nipple–areola complex and the lower lips, moves as a rigid body with the cycling motion of the mandible, while the posterior section of the tongue undulates in a pattern similar to a propagating peristaltic wave, which is essential for swallowing.'* So the tongue moves *with* the lower jaw, lifting to compress the breast/areolar tissue and dropping to create negative pressure with each 'suck'.

Breastfeeding by a mother living with HIV would not be safe if the baby had undergone surgery resulting in bleeding or open wounds in his mouth. In spite of this, mothers have been known to come under pressure to have their baby's tongue-tie divided.

Mothers who need to be cautious about frenotomy should be reassured that it shouldn't be necessary if they can answer 'yes' to two questions:

- Can the baby's tongue extend over the lower gum?
- Can the baby swallow?

While images in textbooks and on the internet show that the tongue can be tethered at the tip (called an anterior tongue tie), I have examined over 3,000 infant oral anatomies and have never seen a newborn's tongue so tethered or tight that it cannot extend over the baby's lower gum. Nor can it prevent a baby latching, or swallowing, or be a contributory factor to sore nipples or low breastmilk supply for the mother. Certainly mothers can experience these problems, but in my experience, the cause is not tongue-tie. Furthermore, the tongue does grow. Unless there is a severe anterior tie, then the recommendation would be to take extra care during positioning and latching. Leave any decision about having your baby undergo a frenotomy to divide a tongue-tie (if indeed there is one) until he is weaned. If you seek professional advice about a tie, then do make sure that any advice is given from the perspective of breastfeeding with HIV.

Nipple shields

Use of a nipple shield, a thin silicone teat which covers the nipple and areola, can be helpful to assist breastfeeding when it would otherwise seem to be impossible. It can be used as a last resort, when all other strategies have failed, for example for:

- short, flat or inverted nipples
- providing a firm super-stimulus to the palate if a non-latching baby can't seem to find the softer, shorter nipple
- assisting milk transfer, by keeping a baby sucking
- keeping the tongue down if a baby is tongue-sucking (suspect this if the baby's cheeks draw inwards with every suck and if you try drawing the nipple back you realise that the baby wasn't attached to the breast at all)
- sore or abraded nipples by providing a glove-like barrier between the nipple and the baby's tongue.

A mother may need to use a shield for only one or two breastfeeds, or for several months. To use a shield:

- it should be stretched over the nipple and areola
- it can be held in place during breastfeeding by the index finger and thumb, with the rest of the fingers supporting the breast as if it is being 'poured' into the shield
- the tip of the shield should be pointed up along the palate for latching, and then the whole teat part should be taken deep into the baby's mouth
- the breast and shield will usually need to be supported well throughout the feed
- the cross-cradle, or football hold may be the easiest position to use for breastfeeding with a shield. Watch for swallowing and ensure that *at the end of the feed there is milk in the shield*, demonstrating that the breast was letting down and that the baby was receiving milk
- when the baby stops breastfeeding, you should check that

the breast has been well drained, and if not, you should hand express or pump the milk left in the breast. This is particularly important in the first days of using a shield and/or as milk production is at peak synthesis, between days 4–9 after the birth (see Chapter 12).

Great care needs to be taken to ensure that the shield doesn't aggravate the nipple damage, either because the holes at the end of the shield abrade the nipples even more, or if the baby takes a short latch on the shield, which can pinch the tip of the nipple, preventing milk transfer and causing even more pain.

Weaning off the shield can be attempted once breastfeeding is going well, the baby is latching easily, and he is getting enough milk to be satisfied.

- choose a time where you know that the baby will be happy
- begin the breastfeed in the normal way
- once the baby is sucking and swallowing well, quickly:
- take the baby off the breast
- remove the shield
- offer the breast without the shield
- the baby should latch and continue sucking
- finish the feed without the shield
- reward the baby with big smiles – this is a big accomplishment
- if your baby becomes upset, re-latch with the shield and try again another time, or another day. Increasing an infant's hunger does not improve sucking skills! The baby is more likely to breastfeed direct when he is happy, well-fed and relaxed.

Resting the nipples

Mothers experiencing sore nipples sometimes ask about 'resting' the nipples, i.e. not breastfeeding direct for a few days, in order to give a damaged nipple time to heal. Either one or both nipples can be rested. While the usual advice is not to stop breastfeeding directly except as an absolute last resort, and instead to revisit positioning and attachment techniques and continue breastfeeding even with damaged or abraded nipples, this is not appropriate in the context of HIV where you want to avoid any possibility of the baby ingesting any of the mother's blood. Instead, it is preferable to temporarily stop breastfeeding, and to express or pump the breasts and feed the expressed breastmilk by cup, spoon or bottle (see Chapter 13). For comfort-sucking, offer your baby your clean finger, pad side up, or a dummy/pacifier. Be sure to keep the affected breast(s) very well drained to maintain your milk supply, and return to breastfeeding direct as soon as possible.

Unlatching

If you must unlatch your baby from the breast, don't just pull away – a baby with a strong suck will hang on and this risks nipple damage. Slide your little finger down beside your nipple, into his mouth and between his gums to break the suction.

Do you need more help?

Breastfeeding is often quite difficult. Sometimes it can seem as if you need six pairs of hands to latch one inexperienced newborn to the breast, and there is nothing wrong with asking for help. One of the difficulties you have, as the mother, is that you can only see the top of your breast and the near side of your baby's face; you can't see underneath, so having another pair of eyes can help. Or you can try latching in front of a mirror.

Many mothers battle with breastfeeding when learning all by themselves. Apparently 80% of them give it up before they are ready. If you try something you've seen or heard about that doesn't work for you, ask for more help, or search the internet or find another video for more ideas. If you search 'breastfeeding help' you can come up with 350 million hits in half a second. There is an answer and a solution that will work somewhere out there! IBCLCs are experienced in solving these kinds of difficulties.

Meanwhile you can ask your partner or an experienced friend to watch what you're doing and see if they can identify the problem;

sometimes a husband or partner can be your extra eyes and hands (see Chapter 6).

If someone else provides hands-on help to latch your baby tor your breast, they should:

- wash their hands thoroughly before they touch you or your baby. (Lactation consultants will usually wear gloves).
- sit beside you and on whichever side is easiest to observe where your baby's *lower jaw* goes on to the breast.
- support the underside of your breast with his/her thumb and place the index and other fingers on top of the breast. Importantly, note that by moving the thumb or fingers slightly, it is possible to cause the nipple to point up, down, or to one side or the other. The nipple should point up on latching and then be released so that it can stretch into the baby's mouth.
- your helper's other hand should hold the baby's body close to your breast, with their palm on the baby's upper back, and the finger and thumb spread wide and placed below and behind the baby's ears. Ensure that your helper doesn't touch the back of your baby's head.
- as explained, anything touching the baby's cheek will stimulate the baby to turn towards it, so you want nothing touching the baby's face at all.
- your helper should tickle the baby's lips with the nipple, wait until he gapes wide, like a yawn, and bring the baby on to the breast.
- on latching, the nipple should be pointed up to touch the baby's palate. The baby should then latch with more of the underside of the areola in the mouth than the top and the helper needs to release pressure of the index finger on the top of the breast to enable the nipple to slide to the back of the baby's throat.
- The helper should check underneath the breast to see that the baby has not sucked in the lower lip. If he has, it can be gently peeled out so that it is 'flanged' against the breast.
- your helper should check that there is no stretching of the

skin, in and out as the baby sucks. If there is, bring the baby's mouth closer to stop the skin stretching. Adjust the baby's or the breast's position so that it stops.
- once the baby is sucking and swallowing well then you can take over – support the breast and the baby yourself and allow the baby to breastfeed for as long as he wants.
- babies learn very fast. Once he has been shown what to do even once or twice, you will find that he is much easier to latch and you will be able to manage by yourself without help.

Getting professional help

You probably wouldn't dream of giving birth by yourself, yet somehow we think that we should know how to breastfeed all on our own. However, we know that breastfeeding is not instinctive, but an extremely complex, learned behaviour. In an ideal world, you would be able to receive individualised help and guidance as you initiate breastfeeding after birth from an IBCLC or experienced breastfeeding counsellor. Ideally this would be one-to-one, face-to-face assistance tailored to your individual situation. After hospital discharge you would receive home visits to check that breastfeeding is still going well, which would include answers to the many questions mothers have when learning to breastfeed a newborn. But we haven't reached this kind of ideal situation yet in the UK or in most other First World countries.

If you're struggling to latch your baby, or if breastfeeding is becoming painful, it's a good idea to consider asking for professional assistance. You can find an IBCLC through Lactation Consultants of Great Britain (LCGB).[12] You can arrange a hospital or home visit for face-to-face help, or an e-consult online. An IBCLC will be able to:

- perform a breast exam
- make an infant oral exam
- undertake a nursing exam to see what your baby is doing at the breast
- tailor information and give help with latching techniques

- provide other recommendations and develop a care plan tailored specifically to:
  - > your unique breast and nipple shape (size, consistency, elasticity)
  - > your baby's oral anatomy (tongue, palate)
- answer your questions and provide reassurance that breastfeeding is going well.

14. BREASTFEEDING PROBLEMS: SUPPLEMENTING, SUSPENDING AND TRANSITIONING BACK

Preventive care

If you've been able to follow the suggestions in earlier chapters, especially those in chapters 6 and 7 about how to initiate breastfeeding and how to manage your breastmilk supply to conserve the milk-producing cells in the breasts, then hopefully the information in this chapter will never be needed. However, not everyone gets off to a good start with breastfeeding. And, with the best will in the world, mothers can face other difficulties and unexpected challenges which mean that exclusive breastfeeding is compromised. This chapter is included so that a mother living with HIV can put into place strategies to protect her baby's nutrition and to preserve or increase breastmilk production should the baby not be able to breastfeed for any reason, or should her milk production fall below what the baby needs.

Breast refusal (nursing strike)

When a baby stops wanting to breastfeed and suddenly refuses the breast for no apparent reason, we call this a 'nursing strike'. A strike is always very distressing. The baby is clearly hungry but he will not breastfeed. The mother is worried that the baby will starve, and she feels rejected when he arches and screams at the breast in spite of her best efforts.

Strikes usually occur from 4–7 months, but they can occur at any time. Mothers often wonder if perhaps the baby is weaning? However, the difference between weaning and a strike is that weaning is gradual but a strike comes on suddenly, accelerating from occasional turning away from the breast to total refusal within 2–3 days.

Strikes often demonstrate that the baby's trust has been broken, for example:

- Babies who have been unusually easy-going may just suddenly dig in their heels and refuse to breastfeed, and the mother may only realise much later that she has been too busy to give enough attention to the baby, or has asked him/her to wait too long, too often for breastfeeds.
- There may have been something unusual happening at home, e.g. visitors coming to stay, or the family may have been away on holiday.
- An older baby may have bitten the nipple and the mother's reaction frightened him.
- The mother may have changed her perfume or deodorant recently, and the baby objects.
- The baby may have recently had a vaccination.
- Sometimes the cause cannot be identified immediately, but may become apparent to the mother later, once the strike is over.

Whatever the cause, various strategies can be tried to resolve a nursing strike:

1. Feed the baby. Express or pump your milk and feed it to the baby by bottle, but *do not attempt to force the baby to breastfeed;* offer, yes, but force, no. Do everything to keep baby happy and calm. If the baby will only accept EBM by bottle or spoon or cup for now, that's fine. If the baby is over six months, you can offer other foods and liquids too, or safe finger foods. Babies who are striking will be hungry and thirsty, and will accept something. EBM would be the best food!
2. Drain the breasts. Keep pumping or expressing to keep the breasts thoroughly and regularly drained to maintain breastmilk production and provide breastmilk to feed to the baby in another way.
3. Treat the situation as a crisis. Friends and family can be called upon to help as they would in any other crisis. Unload all other responsibilities for several days in order to devote 24 hours a day to the baby. Ask friends and relations if they can help look after

other children, do the school run, help with shopping, walk the dog and help with meals and housework.
4. Get back in touch with the baby to help regain his trust, even if these measures seem extreme; hold him all the time, wear him all day e.g. in a sling while you're doing your housework, carry him on your hip, play with him a lot, bath with him, sleep with him, facilitate lots of skin-to-skin and body contact in an attempt to literally get back 'in touch'.
5. *Keep offering the breast, but don't force.* If the baby starts to struggle / arch / cry, stop offering, smile, laugh, pretend you didn't mean it, and when the baby is happy and relaxed again (in an hour or so), offer again. When offering the breast:
   > make sure there are no clothes in the way
   > mother and baby are alone (no distractions, TV, other children, etc) in a quiet darkened room (or in the bath)
   > offer the 'favourite' breast first, in the 'favourite' position, in the 'favourite' place
   > try nursing while standing or rocking the baby. Some babies become enraged if placed horizontal, so the mother needs to slide the baby down from her shoulder and offer the breast with the baby upright. Sometimes having the baby upright straddling her leg can also work
   > 'play' at dabbing the baby's lips with the nipple, taking it away, dabbing again, laughing, keeping everything light and happy, as if this is a big game
   > pretend you are 'charming' the baby: do all the things that he likes, keep him very happy, show him you love him and *keep offering the breast!*
   > the key to success seems to be in persuading the baby that taking the breast is light, fun, normal and safe – above all, he needs to know that he is in control. The mother offers, but it is the baby who has the power to accept or not; the mother needs to regain the baby's trust. This is hard, and sobering for the mother, but she can do it, and what baby could resist this kind of charm offensive for long?

> sleeping with the baby, offering the breast once he is already asleep (sometimes the baby will take it and then wake up, realise what he is doing and reject it again)
> eliminating all perfumes, deodorants
> eliminating possible food sensitivities (e.g. dairy and beef products, other foods that the mother may dislike, caffeine-containing foods/drinks etc)

6. Don't let your frustration show; the baby's refusal will be very distressing, but you must try not to show it – if your feelings become overwhelming, put your baby down somewhere safe, go outside and scream or kick something, but hide this reaction from the baby (easier said than done, but you are bigger, cleverer, smarter than he is).
7. As the strike resolves, and the baby starts to respond to your charm offensive, he will try taking an experimental suck at the breast. He may take one or two swigs and then come off. You should reward the baby with big smiles and congratulations for even the smallest attempt, and let him call the shots, i.e. let him stop when he wants to, and offer again later. Tiny swigs may start to become small sucking bursts. Eventually the baby is willing to breastfeed. When this happens the mother should offer the breast a lot, at every excuse, before she can start to relax and realise that the strike is over.
8. At this point, mothers often realise what went wrong in the first place, and become determined not to let it happen again – i.e. they become much more 'careful' mothers of this quite sensitive baby.
9. These measures are invariably successful. Often the strike is over within hours, not days. But the longer it took to happen, the longer it is likely to take to resolve. Sometimes the mother is not willing to give everything up for the baby, even for a few days, and uses the situation to wean him.
10. If the strike is not over within 3–4 days, consider contacting your IBCLC for more strategies to help resolve the strike as soon as possible. Continue to feed the baby expressed breastmilk by

bottle as described in Chapter 10 until he can be persuaded to resume breastfeeding.

Supplementing the HIV-exposed breastfed baby

'Not enough milk' is the second most common reason that mothers abandon breastfeeding. The mother living with HIV is particularly challenged if her baby fails to thrive on exclusive breastfeeding because the advice from the baby's paediatrician will usually be to start formula supplements in order to protect his nutritional needs. Since the infant feeding recommendation in the context of HIV is for either exclusive breastfeeding or exclusive formula-feeding, this advice effectively translates to exclusive formula-feeding because practising mixed feeding is not recommended due to the increased risk of transmission of the virus. Thus, in practical terms, the need for supplements means that breastfeeding will have to be abandoned. This is heart-breaking for a mother who has had her heart set on breastfeeding.

But all is not lost. There are several questions that can have a bearing on whether supplements are really necessary, and if so, whether mother and baby have to give up breastfeeding:

- Firstly, check the baby's weight to identify whether or not there really is a problem.
- In low weight gain, how serious is the deficit in breastmilk production?
- What strategies can be used to increase the mother's breastmilk supply?
- If supplements are really needed, what, how much, and when should they be offered?
- Does breastfeeding have to be abandoned?
- Can pasteurised mother's own milk be safely fed to the baby with formula supplements?
- Once the baby is gaining weight well, how can the supplements be reduced and then eliminated?
- How can a mother safely transition back to direct breastfeeding?

Answering these questions can suggest a way forward. Various strategies are possible. They will take ingenuity, patience and perseverance, but they can be done! This chapter is written to suggest various simultaneously possible interventions for:

- maintaining breastfeeding
- increasing a mother's breastmilk production and
- feeding/supplementing a low-weight-gain HIV-exposed baby of less than six months of age so that his rate of weight gain normalises
- resuming breastfeeding once the baby has achieved a catch-up gain

Enlisting the help of your healthcare team

Low weight gain can affect your baby's health, so it is strongly advised that:

- Your baby should be under the care of a paediatrician who will monitor your baby's health and provide medical care while you work to increase his breastmilk intake and provide supplements of expressed breastmilk (EBM) or infant formula, as necessary. It may be that the baby's low gain is due to an infection or other health condition that will need treatment before he will start to regain any lost weight.
- You may also need medical advice, special tests and/or prescription drugs from your own HIV clinician or GP.
- It will be helpful to consult an IBCLC or experienced, knowledgeable, skilled breastfeeding counsellor in order to receive face-to-face assistance; to go through your breastfeeding history and to review positioning and latching techniques, in order to tailor a specific breastfeeding care plan for you and your baby.
- Breastfeeding in the context of HIV deserves special care. If you haven't done so already, you should disclose your HIV status to the members of your medical team so that they can make appropriate recommendations in your situation.

'Not enough milk': is there really a problem?

In the newborn period it's fairly common for a baby to experience latching difficulties, or to be sleepy, so that he is not breastfeeding at all. If this happens:

- start expressing your colostrum or early milk on to a spoon and spoon-feed him these tiny quantities every 2–3 hours day and night.
- Often just a teaspoon or two of expressed breastmilk will keep his blood-sugar levels within the normal range, and perk up a sleepy baby enough to become more demanding.
- Frequent little feeds of expressed breastmilk will keep a non-latching baby calm enough to enable you to keep trying him at the breast, whereas leaving him hungry will seriously undermine his breastfeeding skills.
- Feed him the quantities of colostrum/breastmilk shown below, and check his weight to ensure he doesn't lose more than 7% of his birthweight. From day to day you can check his urine and stool output against the figures shown in Chapter 7.

For a baby older than 7–10 days, the belief that you may not be making enough milk can be real, or perceived (i.e. just a needless worry). It's important to distinguish an imagined problem from actual low gain. From day to day you can monitor your baby's urine and stool output to see if he is getting enough milk. If so, in each 24 hours he will produce:

- 6–8 wet nappies (five heavy disposable nappies) with clear urine and
- 3–5 yellow seedy stools

However, looking at wees and poos can be a somewhat subjective observation. The only objective way to tell is to weigh the baby, get out your calculator and check whether he is gaining weight as well as he should, from birth, and from his last weight check.

Weights

Babies who are thriving and obtaining sufficient breastmilk should lose and gain weight at the following rates:

- Loss of up to 7% of birthweight by day three is normal
    > *except* if you received IV fluids during labour, which causes extra newborn weight loss as the baby has an increased urine output in the first 24 hours; if this is the case, then count the weight at 24 hours as the 'birth weight' and compute the difference between 24 hours and three days as the normal newborn weight loss
    > Weight loss of 10% or more demands investigation and recommendations to enhance intake
    > To assess the baby's rate of gain in the next few weeks, calculate from *the lowest weight ever recorded*, not his birthweight
- Thereafter, *as a rule of thumb*, a full-term, healthy baby should regain and gain at the following minimum rates; healthy babies who are breastfeeding well often gain much more:
    > Regain birthweight within 10–14 days (three weeks at most)
    > 0–3 months: 30g/day
    > 3–6 months: 20g/day
    > 6–12 months: 15g/day
- The baby should double his/her birthweight by 4–5 months
- The baby should triple his/her birthweight by one year.

Weight charts showing growth percentiles can be found on the WHO website, where there are growth charts for boys[1] and girls.[2] Your baby's weight can be plotted on the chart, placing his birthweight on the left-hand side.

Mothers in the UK may be urged not to weigh their babies too often, and in particular not to weigh them more than once a month from two weeks to six months of age.[3] This misses the fragile window period for breastfeeding initiation and consolidation which takes place in the first six weeks. Mothers are also sometimes falsely reassured that as long as the baby is gaining some weight he is fine, or that he is 'following his own curve'. Both these situations are misleading because a small deficit in weight gain (due to insufficient milk intake) is very easy to remedy if it is identified in time, but it becomes challenging if low weight gain continues on and on without anyone noticing until suddenly there is a panic at six or 10 weeks.

Weighing your young baby weekly can reassure you that he is doing well on exclusive breastfeeding – or identify if he needs a little more encouragement to take more milk. The baby should follow the percentile for his birth weight and, if he hasn't, something needs to change.

For example, a baby boy weighing 3kg at birth, just above the 15th percentile on the chart, should remain just above the 15th percentile at six weeks and should then weigh approximately 4.5kg.

Low weight gain

In the case of actual low gain, it is helpful if your clinic or Health Visitor will agree to weigh your baby more often than the Royal College of Paediatricians currently recommend, so that you can closely monitor how effective your attempts to increase your breastmilk supply are. Try and weigh the baby naked and always on the same scales, since scales can vary so much. It is the *difference* between one weight and another which tells you the most.

Inadequate weight gain has many causes.[4] Ideally breastfeeding difficulties should be assessed by a Lactation Consultant or breastfeeding specialist, *and the baby should be under medical care* (e.g. a paediatrician) so that his nutrition and health can be monitored while the cause is found and addressed.

Whatever the cause, however, low weight gain shows that the baby has not been taking enough milk, often due to infrequent or too short breastfeeding episodes *for this particular baby*. If this poor situation continues too long the baby may be described as 'failure to thrive' (FTT). This description has no universally accepted definition. In the UK it is described as 'faltering growth'. Infants are generally considered to be failing to thrive (and will usually need to receive supplemental feeding) when their weight drops below the third percentile or is two standard deviations below the mean on a standardised growth chart.[5]

Finding the cause of low gain

Most FTT is not caused by a physical problem, although a check-up to rule out any infection or other health condition in *the baby* is essential. A urinary tract or gastrointestinal tract infection can cause low gain even though, if a baby is breastfed, he may not *seem* sick. Sometimes there can be something more serious which needs treatment. This is why, in any case of low gain, your baby should be checked by your paediatrician. Other medical conditions in *the mother*, like retained placenta, low thyroid levels or drugs such as hormonal contraceptives (see below) can have a negative effect on breastmilk production. Before you start working to increase your milk supply, you should seek an appointment to discuss these possibilities with your doctor who will be able to order lab tests to rule out any problem.

More usually, however, mothers with babies who have failed to gain weight well frequently describe a history of postpartum engorgement having been badly managed, with consequent breast damage and down-regulation of breastmilk production.[6] The unnecessary consequence, as evidenced by the very low breastfeeding rates in the UK, is the mother's realisation that her baby will need formula supplements and the beginning of a slow spiral to complete weaning from the breast in favour of bottle-feeding. Yet very often supplementation of breastfeeding is possible to protect the baby's nutrition while the mother works to increase her breastmilk supply. Sometimes a single cause of low weight gain is never found, but after the problem has resolved the mother may be able to see a combination of small events that led to her baby not gaining weight well, and she will know how to avoid a recurrence with this baby – and with subsequent babies.

Much advice directed at mothers ignores these basic needs of

BREASTFEEDING PROBLEMS

small babies, resulting in inadequate breastmilk intake by the baby, low weight gain and – if not recognised in time – eventual failure to thrive. Causes of low weight gain which are often overlooked are:

- *Infrequent breastfeeds:* most healthy babies need to breastfeed 10–20 times in 24 hours.
- *Limited feeding duration:* most small babies need to breastfeed with active swallowing for 10–40 minutes at each feed, until they have had enough (as indicated by gradually relaxing and falling asleep at the breast); many babies like to cluster-feed on and off for 2–3 hours, particularly in the evenings, and then sleep for 2–3 hours; use of a dummy may limit the time spent at the breast, resulting in inadequate breast drainage which suppresses the mother's milk supply.
- *Hormonal contraceptive use:* women living with HIV are often pressured to use early hormonal contraception shortly after the birth of their babies. Some women find that the progestin-only pill, as well as the combined oral contraceptive pill and injectables, implants, patches or intrauterine devices (IUDs) cause their babies to become much more fussy and demanding than usual,[7] indicating a possible negative effect on the fat/protein content of their breastmilk and/or its quantity.
- *Retained placenta:* if your breasts have never seemed very full since the birth, or your milk has completely failed to come in, then this should be examined as a cause of any apparently unexplained low weight gain in the first six weeks after birth.[8] You will need to seek urgent medical advice and possibly receive an ultrasound scan to rule out this possibility and treatment if this is the cause.
- *Severe postpartum haemorrhage:* this can inhibit full breastmilk production until the mother's haemoglobin levels (Hb) return to normal; the mother's Hb should be checked, and she may receive iron supplements as she recovers, which may take as long as six weeks.
- *Mother's thyroid function:* this should be assessed in any case of

'not enough milk' if there is no other obvious cause.[9]
- *Theca-luteinising cysts or polycystic ovarian syndrome:* should be considered if the mother's milk fails to 'come in' within the first few days after birth.[10]
- *Inadequate glandular breast tissue:* an unlikely cause of lactation failure, but should be considered if there have been no breast changes during pregnancy, if the breasts are very widely spaced and/or there is a variation in size, with puffy areolas.
- *Sore nipples:* the cause should be assessed and addressed (see Chapter 13) – and may be due either to poor positioning and attachment of the baby at the breast, or a bacterial infection, or (less likely) a fungal infection; the pain may be so severe that the mother is unwilling to keep the baby at breast long enough for him to obtain enough milk.
- *Tongue-tie* is frequently cited as a cause of sore nipples and/or inadequate milk transfer, but this *is the least likely cause;* other causes should be looked for and addressed first before it can be concluded that anterior or posterior tongue-tie and/or upper labial or buccal tie is a cause of sore nipples, or low weight gain/failure to thrive. Frenotomy to divide the tie(s) would require an HIV-exposed baby to be taken off the breast and fed pasteurised expressed breastmilk to avoid possible contact of the baby's bloodstream with the virus until healing has taken place. Following frenotomy, the baby who is gaining poorly *should continue to be followed up* to ascertain that the procedure has been effective in reversing the previous low gain and to ensure that it was not due to another undiagnosed cause.

Babies who are consistently receiving inadequate intake may show certain classic behaviours or characteristics:

- In the newborn period there may be *prolonged jaundice,* the *baby loses >10% of his/her birthweight in the first three days of life* and *does not regain the lost weight by 10–14 days of age.*
- *Dark urine and scanty or no stools* (as outlined above) – babies who

are getting enough milk produce 6–8 wet nappies with clear urine and 3–5 yellow, mustard stools in each 24 hours. After 6–8 weeks some babies produce fewer stools and if intake is very low they produce fewer wet nappies too. If they continue to gain well, fewer stools can be considered normal, but if the weight gain falters, it can be concluded that there is inadequate intake.

- *Low or no weight gain:* many healthcare personnel, as well as friends, and social media groups, will offer false reassurance that low gain in a breastfed baby is normal, but it is not; all cases of consistently inadequate gain lasting more than a couple of weeks should be fully investigated and only if there is no other identified cause, and if the baby is pronounced fit, healthy and developing normally by his paediatrician, should a mother be persuaded to feel complacent about her baby's low weight gain. In the meantime, she should breastfeed more often and for longer using breast compression to assist the baby's milk intake.
- At first, the hungry baby shows *prolonged and frequent crying,* which is often mistaken for colic/gas/wind, or the baby is pacified/soothed with a dummy.
- Later, the hungry *baby may want to feed all day and sleep all night;* well-meaning friends and advisors may inappropriately endorse either of these abnormal situations by either urging the mother to continue breastfeeding 'on demand', and by offering congratulations that the baby is sleeping through the night; and the mother may also reason that because she is feeding the baby all day, and he is sleeping all night, that he must be getting enough. The truth, however, is that the baby becomes so exhausted by attempting and failing to obtain enough nourishment during the day that he is too tired to wake up often enough to breastfeed adequately at night. Long intervals without drainage will deplete his mother's breastmilk supply still further.
- During breastfeeding, it may be observed that there is a *very short period of swallowing;* thereafter the baby wants to stay

attached to the breast, but *mostly flutter-sucks with closed eyes,* and he wakes again to protest and show hunger only when taken off the breast.
- The low gain or FTT baby usually has *high muscle tone;* he seems very strong and wiry, keeping his elbows tight to his body, unlike the well-fed baby who will gradually relax during breastfeeding, uncurl his hands and fall into a deep sleep; at the same time, the baby starts to become very *watchful,* and his *face may look like a little old man.*
- Mothers of low gain babies are sometimes falsely reassured that the baby is still growing in length. However, 'stunting' (when a child fails to grow taller) is a very late stage of under-nutrition; most often the baby continues to grow in length but there is 'wasting' (loss of body fat, then muscle mass) for some time before it affects the baby's growth. So the baby who is not getting enough to eat *may continue to grow in length, but his/her skin looks too loose,* especially on the buttocks, arms and thighs. Because the baby is usually well-covered most of the time, and/or because parents are with the baby every day, and/or may be in denial, this gradual deterioration may first be noticed by a friend, a grandparent or a healthcare provider.

Baby's intake

The baby who is not 'getting enough' at the breast (as evidenced by consistently inadequate weight gain), needs to receive help to breastfeed as effectively as possible and often supplementation, preferentially, as follows

- First choice: breastfeeding direct, at breast
- Second choice: mother's expressed breastmilk, if available
- Third choice: infant formula

Are supplements really necessary?

A baby who is growing well on breastfeeding alone doesn't need supplementation. However, if a baby is not gaining quite enough, a mother can try to increase her breastmilk production and the baby's intake as follows.

At each feed:

1. Breastfeed for 20–30 minutes in total (15 minutes each breast), using breast compression to increase swallowing.
2. Switch breasts as necessary when breast compression no longer results in more sucking/swallowing bursts.
3. Stop after a maximum of 30 minutes.
4. Feed any previously expressed breastmilk as a top-up.
5. Settle the baby (allow the baby to go to sleep).
6. As soon as possible after feeding, express any milk that the baby has left behind, to save for supplementing by bottle later.
7. Breastfeed again after an interval of 60–90 minutes.
8. This means that the baby will be fed with maximum intake at least 10 times in 24 hours.

If these measures don't result in an increased rate of gain within a short period, then – with the paediatrician's advice – the mother will probably need to start formula supplements to protect the baby's nutrition.

How much to supplement?

While continuing to increase your own breastmilk production, you can work out how far below his ideal weight the baby is and offer supplements proportionally to top up to the total amount he needs every day, e.g. a baby who is gaining only half the amount of desired weight could be offered half the 24 hour total as a supplement. A baby who is not breastfeeding effectively (or at all) and/or fails to start gaining weight after just a week or two of extra feeding will require the following *total* amounts of milk in 24 hours:

Day 1: 60ml/kg/day
Day 2: 90ml/kg/day
Day 3: 120ml/kg/day

Day 4 – Day 10: 150ml/kg/day
Day 10 onwards: 180ml/kg/day

- If you need to start feeding the baby extra formula supplements, then it is important to *stop breastfeeding and use pasteurised expressed breastmilk instead.*
- Babies who are recovering from failure to thrive (very low/ no gain over an extended period) may become extremely 'demanding' and may easily take increasing quantities once they have the energy to stay awake longer and to indicate hunger.
- Generally it is better to allow the baby more supplements rather than trying to limit them. In consultation with the baby's paediatrician it may be appropriate to feed the baby up to 280–300ml/kg/day (i.e. any EBM and formula top-ups, by bottle) while he achieves a 'catch-up gain'.
- It's important for the mother not to feel too discouraged if she realises that her milk was far below what her baby needed – it *can* be increased while the baby achieves a catch-up gain and then his appetite drops down to a more normal intake.
- Once the baby has reached the weight he should be on his percentile for his age, then he will usually become less demanding and will be satisfied with the quantities set out above, e.g. 180ml/kg/day.
- Experience shows that it usually takes as long for low weight gain to be resolved as it took to happen (another reason for weighing your baby weekly to identify a small, easy-to-fix problem promptly).

Caution about formula supplementation

In the context of breastfeeding with HIV, as soon as infant formula is given to the baby younger than six months then the mother should:

- *take the baby off the breast and stop all direct breastfeeding*
- *express or pump her milk very often, at least 8–10 times in each*

24 hours – this is to:
> drain the breasts and increase milk production, and
> feed the baby the expressed milk
- store and *pasteurise* the milk before feeding it to the baby (see Chapter 11)
- feed the baby her own pasteurised breastmilk and top-up with formula to the amount the baby needs
- continue using pasteurised breastmilk
   > for the whole time that the baby receives formula supplements (to avoid 'mixed feeding')
   > AND, *for three weeks past the time that formula supplements are no longer necessary, to allow the baby's gut to heal from any damage caused by the formula, before returning to direct exclusive breastfeeding.*

Method of delivering supplements

EBM or formula supplements can be fed to the baby as follows:

- By cup
- By spoon
- By finger-feeding
- By bottle

Note: mothers are often encouraged to offer supplements at the breast through the use of a supplemental nursing system. If the baby is receiving formula, this would not be appropriate in the context of HIV.

Supplementation in itself will not decrease breastmilk production

Mothers are often advised that supplementation with formula in a bottle will decrease their breastmilk supply, but this need not necessarily happen as long as they maximise breastmilk production by pumping and expressing very often. The breasts need to be kept very well drained to be stimulated to make more milk.

Breastmilk synthesis is faster, the emptier the breast. The fat content of breastmilk is also higher, the emptier the breast. Thus 'saving' the milk in the breasts so that the baby can have 'a good feed' several hours later is counterproductive. Instead, draining the breasts often – even if they seem fairly empty – will increase your breastmilk production in the fastest possible way.[11]

Mothers living with HIV are also often persuaded that they must either breastfeed or bottle-feed and that it is not worth continuing to work towards resuming breastfeeding if the amount of breastmilk produced is quite small; this is not true. Breastmilk is so valuable to the baby that even 50ml/day will keep him healthier than none; in addition, breastmilk production can nearly always be increased with a view to replacing the supplement.

As the baby's nutrition improves so will his energy; once he has reached the appropriate weight he should have been for his age, then he will almost certainly be able to breastfeed effectively, *but probably not before* – while he is still catching up on his weight he may still need extra bottle-feeding, preferably breastmilk. If there is not enough EBM, then formula supplements will be needed as well. It may take quite some time to resolve a low weight gain/failure to thrive difficulty, but if a mother is motivated enough to put in the time and hard work of expressing her milk and pasteurising it, and supplementing with only enough formula as needed, then the rewards are very great.

In addressing the problem of inadequate breastmilk intake in the context of HIV, there are only a few basic rules:

- Feed the baby as much breastmilk as possible and, if necessary, extra formula
- Drain the breasts frequently
- Pasteurise the breastmilk to avoid the risks associated with 'mixed feeding'
- Enlist help with other household tasks and, except for feeding and caring for the baby, rest as much as possible
- Eat well, but you do not need any special foods, biscuits or herbs
- Drink to thirst (too much fluid can decrease milk production)

- Seek medical advice about whether your doctor would be willing to prescribe a galactagogue such as domperidone[12] to increase breastmilk production.

The easiest method of feeding the baby enough milk while maximising breastmilk production

Time management when you're working to feed up a baby who has gained inadequate weight is hard, and can seem overwhelming. But with a little organisation it is not too difficult, and in fact when your baby is well-fed and full, rather than having to feed him 'all day long', you may unexpectedly find you have *more* time for other things.

At each feed:
- Feed the baby with any available expressed pasteurised breastmilk
- if necessary top-up to the right amount with formula
- for example: if the baby needs a feed of 60ml, and there is only 20ml expressed pasteurised breastmilk available, feed the EBM first, and then feed 40ml of formula
- Settle the baby (cuddle, comfort, allow the baby to fall asleep in arms with a dummy/pacifier, or sucking your finger, pad side up)
- As soon as possible after feeding, express both breasts at least twice (hand-expression or pump, or both, whichever is most efficient) for a maximum of 10–15 minutes or until there are only small, creamy drops of milk being produced. *The key to milk production is frequent and efficient breast drainage,* so it is important to express to the very last drop! Over time, this – more than anything else – will stimulate the breasts to produce more.
- Store any expressed breastmilk in the fridge; if the quantities are very tiny, then store several batches in the same bottle until you have a reasonable quantity for pasteurising and feeding. It's fine to save all the small amounts and feed them to the baby all at once instead of dividing up them up into several feeds.

- Pasteurise your expressed milk in batches not exceeding 120ml.
- Feed the baby the pasteurised breastmilk first before formula top-ups.
- Do not mix expressed breastmilk and formula in the same bottle – this is to avoid waste in case the baby doesn't finish it all.

Monitoring your progress: keeping a chart of each day's feeds:
Keep a chart of:

- breastmilk feeds
- formula supplements
- the time and amounts of breastmilk expressed
- the baby's urine and stool output. A baby who is getting enough breastmilk should produce 6–8 wet nappies (five disposables) with clear urine in each 24 hours. He should also produce 3–5 yellow, seedy stools. A baby who receives formula supplements may produce fewer darker stools, but should still produce clear urine. If he is not producing this output, feed him more.
- At the end of each day total up the amount and type of pasteurised breastmilk and formula fed to the baby, and the times and amounts of breastmilk that you expressed. These figures can be used over time to assess progress, or to show where something needs to be altered or improved. You would expect the amount of formula supplements to decrease as the amount of breastmilk you can express (and the baby receives) goes up.
- In this way, you can track the baby's intake, and your breastmilk production. It is important to drain the breasts at least 8–10 times in 24 hours, and over time you will see that your breastmilk supply increases and that EBM can then be used to replace formula.

Each week:
- The baby should be weighed.
- Using the chart she keeps, the mother should assess the baby's increasing breastmilk intake and – over time – her success in

reducing the quantity of formula supplements needed for catch-up weight gain and then to maintain adequate weight gain.
- The baby's doctor should be consulted regularly to monitor the baby's health while the mother works on increasing her breastmilk production.

Additional help

Apart from baby-care, the mother should try and rest as much as possible; unload all other responsibilities, accept help from the baby's father, friends, family and neighbours with all other tasks. It may take as long to build up the milk supply as it took to fall below the baby's needs, so the mother will need to be kind to herself, to be prepared to put in the time to express her milk, and to wait for her baby to grow stronger.

The mother should consider discussing with her doctor the advisability of taking a galactagogue to increase breastmilk production. In the UK the most commonly used drug has been domperidone (10mg, three times a day), which was available over the counter in pharmacies, but there is some concern about its use now – the mother should consult her doctor. In southern Africa, the most commonly prescribed galactagogue is sulpiride (50mg three times a day until breastmilk production is sufficient to exclusively feed the baby, then taper off very gradually, e.g. twice a day for a week, then once a day for a week, to avoid a sudden drop in milk production).

The baby should be under the care of an experienced, breastfeeding-friendly GP or paediatrician. It is important to rule out all medical causes of low weight gain, to treat any health conditions in mother and baby, and to continue follow-ups to monitor the baby's nutrition and development. If a doctor advises complete weaning from the breast, then the mother committed to breastfeeding may wish to consider seeking further medical advice or a second opinion from a doctor who has wide experience in working with breastfed babies.

Transitioning back to breastfeeding

Once the baby has taken his last supplemental feed of formula, the mother should continue to feed her baby her pumped and pasteurised breastmilk for a full *three weeks* to give his gut time to heal from the exposure to formula.

After three weeks, she can stop pasteurising and offer raw breastmilk and/or resume direct breastfeeding.

The mother may need to reteach her baby how to breastfeed, using lots of cuddling and holding in between feeding times, and offering the breast often for food and comfort-sucking, but offering bottles of expressed milk to top-up with at first while the baby re-establishes his breastfeeding skills.

As the baby starts swallowing more milk during breastfeeding you can monitor his urine and stool output and continue to weigh weekly to ensure he is taking enough, while cutting down bottles of expressed breastmilk gradually.

Finally, as the baby's strength improves and if his rate of weight gain remains normal, you should be able to maintain breastfeeding and eventually gradually eliminate all expressed breastmilk supplements.

Avoiding nipple confusion

Mothers and their supporters often worry that a breastfed baby who is receiving a bottle will become nipple-confused. However, working to maintain breastfeeding while providing appropriate supplementation is difficult and time-consuming, and it seems logical that the mother should use the easiest, quickest method that she can find of feeding the supplements; this may be by bottle. Almost consistently in these circumstances the baby is happy to resume breastfeeding (when that would be safe) on a 'full' breast, i.e. when the mother's breastmilk supply has increased to the point that she can fully meet his needs. The key seems to be keeping the baby very well fed and during the transition to exclusive direct breastfeeding at the breast to keep bottle-feeds as short as possible, so that there is not much comfort-sucking on the bottle. When transitioning back to the breast offer the breast before the baby becomes too hungry, as well as often between feeds for comfort-sucking, so that the whole mummy-breastfeeding experience becomes once again a happy, enjoyable part of the baby's life.

Measuring success

The first weeks can be discouraging, but if she has expressed and pumped as recommended above, the mother will be able to see from her chart that her breastmilk supply is increasing. Eventually she should be able to gradually reduce the amount of formula supplements by replacing them with breastmilk.

If the baby still requires supplements by the age of six months, then it is safe to stop pasteurising any breastmilk that he is taking, or you can resume direct breastfeeding. Solid foods can gradually replace any formula offered, and the mother can continue breastfeeding with solid foods for as long as she and the baby want.

15. SUPPRESSION OF LACTATION

How the breasts stop making milk

By lengthening the intervals between breastfeeding sessions, or by breastfeeding for shorter times than the baby needs, a mother can inadvertently cause her milk supply to fail, as explained in Chapter 14. By causing the breasts to be inadequately drained, both of these strategies thereby gradually suppress lactation. If not drained out during breastfeeding or pumping, a protein in the milk (called feedback inhibitor of lactation, or FIL) signals the milk-producing cells within the breasts to make less, and then even less. A mother who deliberately wants to suppress lactation can use this information to her advantage.

Reasons behind suppression of lactation

Circumstances in which mothers might be considering lactation suppression include:

- Medical advice not to breastfeed due to the risk of HIV transmission, either from birth, or later[1,2]
- A desire not to breastfeed at all, from birth (i.e. maternal choice)
- Plans for early weaning; to stop breastfeeding after a few days, weeks or months
- Plans to stop breastmilk-feeding by bottle

Drugs to suppress lactation

There are difficult and easy ways to suppress lactation. In the past, a drug called *bromocriptine* was often prescribed for two weeks. It was withdrawn for this purpose[3] because of

- the risk of stroke or even death
- severe side effects such as nausea and dizziness which is so severe that mothers taking it were unable to stand up
- risk of severe postpartum depression due to plummeting

prolactin levels
- replacement by a similar drug called *cabergoline*.

Cabergoline is not reported to have all the dangerous side effects of bromocriptine,[4] though mothers have reported experiencing many similar side effects. It is administered as 1mg in a single dose on the first day post-partum (which may completely inhibit postpartum lactation) or, for the suppression of established lactation, 0.25mg is taken every 12 hours for two days for a total of 1mg. Like bromocriptine, cabergoline suppresses the release of prolactin, and can cause severe depression and a grief reaction.[5] Consequently many mothers prefer not to take it.

Outdated advice

Great care needs to be taken when suppressing lactation. Outdated, inhumane and dangerous myth-information is still handed out. Mothers are still mistakenly advised to:

- 'bind' the breasts with tight cloths or to wear a tight bra
- do nothing to relieve engorgement, even if it is severe, in case reducing over-fullness causes the breasts to go on producing milk
- limit fluid intake in the mistaken belief that dehydration will stop milk production

If engorgement is ignored:

- it is important to know that the breasts can become dangerously overfull within a short space of time, say within six hours (e.g. overnight)
- the breasts will become painfully overfull, then badly engorged; the skin on the breasts becomes stretched and shiny, and the breasts feel hard and 'wooden'
- the mother may get 'milk fever' (the temperature rises in an effort to combat the effects of milk being reabsorbed into the bloodstream and to protect the breasts from infection)

- the milk may taste salty, indicating that the tight junctions between the milk-producing cells have opened, allowing HIV viral levels to rise
- there is pain
- the *sudden* drop in prolactin levels caused by lack of breast stimulation can lead to feelings of depression and grief (the body thinks the baby died)
- there is a real risk of mastitis which, if also ignored, can lead to abscess (see Chapter 12)

Preferred method of suppressing lactation quickly, or from birth

The kindest, easiest way to suppress lactation quickly:

- express a little milk (to comfort) whenever the breasts feel a little overfull
- express no more, and no less milk than you need to, to avoid feeling tight and overfull
- from days 4–9, as the milk comes in, you may need to express very often, then express or pump as often as necessary to avoid becoming overfull – in the first couple of days this may be every 3–4 hours, but as the breasts start to make less milk, so the intervals between needing to pump/express/breastfeed will gradually lengthen and the time that the mother needs to pump for will shorten as the milk being made decreases
- gently massage any lumpy areas down towards the nipple and pump/express again
- in between expressing, tuck fresh, raw, cabbage leaves around the breasts. Cabbage seems to suppress lactation, though the mechanism for this phenomenon has not been fully explained
- down-regulation of milk production will be well underway within four days, and you will usually find that you can lengthen the intervals between needing to express, from about every three hours to every four hours, then five or six hours
- within a week to 10 days you may only need to express 2–3 times in 24 hours

- when you find that you don't need to express for about 24 hours without getting too full, then it is probably safe to stop
- by the end of two weeks you may not need to express again
- It may take six weeks, or even longer, before the breasts completely stop milk production; this is normal
- the breasts may seem soft and flat for several weeks, but as the milk-producing cells involute, fat cells in the breasts gradually replace them, particularly with each monthly cycle of ovulation and menstruation
- mothers who are no longer lactating need to be aware that their fertility will return fairly quickly and seek medical advice about contraception.

Suppressing lactation gradually or later after six months

When a mother who has been breastfeeding for some time wants to stop later, there are several advantages to suppressing lactation very gradually, over the course of several weeks:

- for a mother with HIV, stopping breastfeeding slowly has been shown to be safer for the baby[6]
- gradual milk suppression guards against the breasts becoming too full and reduces the likelihood of elevated viral levels in the milk
- gradual milk suppression allows the baby a longer time to get used to the changeover from breastmilk to a breastmilk-substitute (formula)
- It gives time for the mother to assess that the baby is tolerating formula-feeding
- If there are problems, e.g. digestive or immunological problems (asthma, eczema) gradual weaning allows the mother
  > to slow down the weaning process, or
  > even to stop it altogether, and continue breastfeeding for a while longer

To suppress lactation gradually:

- simply breastfeed or pump a little less often than usual, or breastfeed or pump for slightly shorter times, until the breasts are comfortable, but not fully drained
- drop a breastfeed or pumping session only when you are sure that things are going well. Leaving the breasts just a little too full signals them to make less. Having a week or two between dropping breastfeeds one at a time will slowly reduce lactation while keeping the breasts as healthy as possible
- let the breasts remain just a *little* too full: this signals the milk-producing cells to make a little less milk, and then less still, until you no longer need to express at all, as described above

How to avoid mixed feeding for a baby under six months

A mother living with HIV whose baby is under six months old needs to be careful to avoid mixed feeding (breastfeeding *and* formula-feeding together). Once she starts making the changeover to formula-feeding, she should immediately stop breastfeeding directly. She can feed her expressed breastmilk to the baby once it has been home-pasteurised (see Chapter 11).

Frozen saved breastmilk

If you are saving your expressed breastmilk it can be frozen. However, freezing does not inactivate HIV in the milk; if you will be using it for mixed feeding later, it should be pasteurised first. You can pasteurise it either before or after freezing.

Risk of mastitis

During lactation suppression you need to be very aware of the increased risk of a blocked duct or mastitis. If you develop hard, lumpy, inflamed, painful areas on one or both breasts you should treat as for a blocked duct or mastitis (see Chapter 12):

- stop trying to suppress lactation in the affected breast
- start draining the breast as much and as often as possible (as

described in Chapter 12)
- seek prompt medical advice about the need for an antibiotic *and continue draining the affected breast*
- the risk of breast abscess is very high during weaning with mastitis, and is completely avoidable with good breast care
- home-pasteurise any expressed breastmilk from the affected breast before feeding it to the baby

16. CONCLUSION

An understanding of the basic principles of how breastfeeding works enables a mother living with HIV to decide whether she wants to breastfeed, and if so, how long for. Being familiar with some of the research on HIV and breastfeeding can reassure you about how to avoid unnecessary risks, and enable you to discuss the implications of your wishes with your HIV clinicians.

When considered with existing knowledge of mother and/or infant causes and consequences of breast and nipple pathology, recent research gives us greater insight into factors influencing both maternal HIV infectivity and infant susceptibility to infection during breastfeeding. Most importantly, knowing what these causes might be can suggest how you can avoid them. We now know that exposing the baby's immature gut to infant formula causes damage, so that virus in breastmilk can pass into the baby's bloodstream. Thus it is mixed feeding *before* six months, but *not after* six months which poses a risk of transmission of HIV to the baby. We also know that infectivity of the virus is directly related to viral load. The research is clear that when you, as a mother living with HIV, receive – and take – effective antiretroviral drugs, your viral load is so suppressed that it becomes undetectable on a test. When your baby reaches six months of age with a mature, healthy gut, and you continue to adhere to your ART medications, the chances of him becoming infected through mixed feeding are also virtually zero.

Working with just a few rules of lactation physiology you will be able to initiate breastfeeding and ensure ample milk production so that your baby will need nothing but your own milk for the recommended time of six full months. Working along with the normal rules of breastmilk synthesis, you can take good care of your breasts, and avoid over-fullness, engorgement or mastitis and their sequel, leading to 'the domino effect of lactation failure'.[1] You can suppress your lactation a little or a lot, or you can increase it a little or a lot – in other words, you can manage your own lactation, by yourself. Most successful breastfeeding mothers become aware of this physiology and are able to work along and around it to have a happy breastfeeding experience.

A mother living with HIV who experiences breast or nipple problems, or whose baby gains inadequate weight on breastmilk alone, may be advised to wean her baby completely on to formula since mixed feeding is risky. With good breast self-care, breast and nipple problems are largely preventable or, at the very least, can be much reduced. However, if supplements or substitutes for direct breastfeeding are necessary, it is possible for you to use your own heat-treated or home-pasteurised milk, usually on a temporary basis, as a feasible breastfeeding replacement until you can return to breastfeeding direct.

Eventually, a mother living with HIV will want to wean her baby. You can continue breastfeeding for as long as the baby wants, but this is unusual, and in the context of HIV it usually happens that it is the mother who makes this decision and takes active steps to stop breastfeeding. Weaning after a happy breastfeeding experience is hard for the baby. Ideally, weaning will be done slowly and with great care so that your baby can be helped to replace breastfeeding with other foods and comfort measures. You yourself, as the mother, may also find stopping breastfeeding emotionally and physically painful, but there are ways to make this difficult process easier. If you need to suppress lactation quickly, you can work in reverse with the known principles of breastmilk synthesis to avoid pain and damage to the breasts and the unpleasant side effects of drugs to suppress lactation.

ACKNOWLEDGEMENTS

Writing this book would not have been possible had the mothers and babies I worked with over the last 35 years not been willing to so generously share their breastfeeding journeys with me in the hours, days, weeks, months or even years after giving birth to and then breastfeeding their babies. I want to express my deep admiration and gratitude for their gallantry as they allowed me to walk with them at one of the most sensitive and special times of their lives. Thanks to social media, I am still in touch with many of them today to see how their babies have grown into beautiful young adults, graduating from university, getting married and having their own babies.

A special vote of thanks goes to the hundreds of mothers of low weight gain/failure to thrive babies I have worked with, for their resolve and motivation to maintain breastfeeding and re-establish a full milk supply in very challenging situations; and to their babies, most of whom went on to exclusively breastfeed. I learned so much about lactation management from their histories, and from following them up for so long. It was an invaluable experience, not just in situations where breastfeeding seemed to be about to fail, but in developing strategies to prevent problems in the future.

My gratitude goes to the baby-friendly paediatricians in Harare, Zimbabwe, who not only referred babies to me, but were so knowledgeable about the health benefits of breastfeeding that they were willing to monitor the babies' health while the mothers, babies and I worked to fine-tune and maximise breastfeeding. They were all so generous with the facts, figures and knowledge they shared with me that I could not have wished for better mentors. I have endeavoured to pay their generosity forward by taking what they taught me to other mother-baby pairs in other countries.

Deep appreciation goes to Maureen Minchin, Ted Greiner, James Akre, Jack Newman, Marion Thompson, David Bratt, Regina da Silva, George Kent, Anna Coutsoudis, Penny Reimers, and many others, who have always been so generous with sharing their expertise, opinions, knowledge of breastfeeding and writings over the years.

My love and gratitude go to my husband, Alan, and my clever (formerly breastfed) sons, Ian, Bryn and Shaun, for their patient support and technical skills over the years. They have enabled me firstly to work in a profession I love, and then opened the door for me to a wider world of colleagues and friends out there in cyberspace with whom to communicate, brainstorm and share knowledge and ideas.

Special thanks also go to the mothers living with HIV that I have worked with, who have shared their hopes and dreams of breastfeeding with me and trusted me with their sensitive personal information. Breastfeeding with HIV in a First World country has been made much more difficult by local bottle-feeding norms and what seems like casual exaggeration of the risks of transmission of the virus through breastfeeding. When bottle-feeding is seen to be so normal and so safe, why would you want to expose your baby to the possibility of acquiring HIV through breastfeeding? But the mothers who have their hearts set on nursing their babies, like 'real mothers', are prepared to look past the prejudice and poor practice in order to find the information they need to breastfeed as safely as possible; they keep on searching until they're able to access enough how-to information to succeed; they take their antiretroviral therapy to keep themselves and their babies healthy; they go for their viral load tests and have their babies tested, as advised. They have let me know what worked, what was easy and what was difficult and challenging. They are also such good ambassadors for breastfeeding with their own healthcare personnel. Their stories have made writing this book possible.

REFERENCES

Chapter 1: Introduction
1. HIV and Infant Feeding - A Policy Statement developed collaboratively by UNAIDS, UNICEF and WHO (UNAIDS, 1997, 12 p.) https://www.ncbi.nlm.nih.gov/pubmed/10453706 (accessed 28 March 2020
2. WHO 2009, HIV and infant feeding, Revised Principles and Recommendations. Rapid Advice, November 2009 http://whqlibdoc.who.int/publications/2009/9789241598873_eng.pdf
3. WHO recommendation for exclusive breastfeeding for all babies everywhere https://www.who.int/news/item/15-01-2011-exclusive-breastfeeding-for-six-months-best-for-babies-everywhere
4. UK Infant Feeding Survey 2010, with tables and links https://digital.nhs.uk/data-and-information/publications/statistical/infant-feeding-survey/infant-feeding-survey-uk-2010
5. WABA, Understanding International Policy on HIV and Breastfeeding: A Comprehensive Resource, Second edition, published 14 July 2018 http://waba.org.my/understanding-international-policy-on-hiv-and-breastfeeding-a-comprehensive-resource/
6. Morrison P, HIV and breastfeeding: the untold story Pinter & Martin, London, 2022

Chapter 2: The research on HIV and breastfeeding
1. WHO overview and recommendations on exclusive breastfeeding at https://www.who.int/health-topics/breastfeeding#tab=tab_1
2. WHO 2010. Guidelines on HIV and infant feeding. Principles and recommendations for infant feeding in the context of HIV and a summary of evidence. 1.Breast feeding 2.Infant nutrition 3.HIV infections – in infancy and childhood. 4.HIV infections – transmission. 5.Disease transmission, Vertical – prevention and control. 6.Infant formula. 7.Guidelines. I.World Health Organization. ISBN 978 92 4 159953 5 information available at http://www.who.int/child_adolescent_health/documents/9789241599535/en/index.html
3. Kuhn L, Aldrovandi G. Pendulum Swings in HIV-1 and Infant Feeding Policies: Now Halfway Back. Adv Exp Med Biol. 2012;743:273-87. http://www.ncbi.nlm.nih.gov/pubmed/22454357
4. Ziegler JB, Cooper DA, Johnson RO, Gold J. Postnatal transmission of AIDS-associated retrovirus from mother to infant. Lancet. 1985 Apr 20;i(8434):896-8. https://www.ncbi.nlm.nih.gov/pubmed/2858746
5. UNAIDS 1997, HIV and Infant Feeding - A Policy Statement developed collaboratively by UNAIDS, UNICEF and WHO, https://www.ncbi.nlm.nih.gov/pubmed/10453706
6. WHO 2009, HIV and infant feeding, Revised Principles and Recommendations. Rapid Advice, November 2009 http://whqlibdoc.who.int/publications/2009/9789241598873_eng.pdf
7. Delaney M, History of HAART – the true story of how effective multi-drug therapy was developed for treatment of HIV disease. Retrovirology 2006

Volume 3 Supplement 1, Article S6, https://retrovirology.biomedcentral.com/articles/10.1186/1742-4690-3-S1-S6

8. Coutsoudis A, Pillay K, Spooner E et al (1999). Influence of infant-feeding patterns on early mother-to-child transmission of HIV-1 in Durban, South Africa: a prospective cohort study. Lancet 354(9177):471-6.

9. Coutsoudis A, Pillay K, Kuhn L et al (2001). Method of feeding and transmission of HIV-1 from mothers to children by 15 months of age: prospective cohort study from Durban, South Africa. AIDS 15(3):379-87.

10. Iliff PJ, Piwoz EG, Tavengwa NV et al (2005). Early exclusive breastfeeding reduces the risk of postnatal HIV-1 transmission and increases HIV-free survival. AIDS 19(7):699–708.

11. Palombi L, Marazzi MC, Voetberg A et al. Treatment acceleration program and the experience of the DREAM program in prevention of mother-to-child transmission of HIV. AIDS 2007; 21(Suppl 4):S65–71.

12. Marazzi MC, Nielsen-Saines K, Buonomo E, Scarcella P, Germano P, Majid NA, Zimba I, Ceffa S, Palombi L. Increased Infant Human Immunodeficiency Virus-Type One Free Survival at One Year of Age in Sub-Saharan Africa With Maternal Use of Highly Active Antiretroviral Therapy During Breast-Feeding. Pediatr Infect Dis J 2009;28: 483–487 https://pubmed.ncbi.nlm.nih.gov/19483516/

13. Chibwesha CJ, Giganti MJ, Putta N, Chintu N, Mulindwa J, Dorton BJ, Chi BH, Stringer JS, Stringer EM. Optimal Time on HAART for Prevention of Mother-to-Child Transmission of HIV. J Acquir Immune Defic Syndr. 2011 Oct 1;58(2):224-8. doi: 10.1097/QAI.0b013e318229147e, http://www.ncbi.nlm.nih.gov/pubmed/21709566

14. Shapiro RL, Hughes MD, Ogwu A et al. Antiretroviral regimens in pregnancy and breast-feeding in Botswana. New England Journal of Medicine 2010;362(24):2282–94

15. Homsy J, Moore D, Barasa A et al (2010). Breastfeeding, mother-to-child HIV transmission, and mortality among infants born to HIV-infected women on highly active antiretroviral therapy in rural Uganda. Journal of Acquired Immune Deficiency Syndromes 53(1):28–35.

16. Thomas TK, Masaba R, Borkowf CB et al (2011). Triple-antiretroviral prophylaxis to prevent mother-to-child HIV transmission through breastfeeding -the Kisumu Breastfeeding Study, Kenya: a clinical trial. PLoS Medicine 8(3):e1001015. http://1.usa.gov/1wCtovS [Accessed 23 October 2014

17. Ngoma MS, Misir A, Wilboard M, Rampakakis E, Sampalis JS, Elong a, Chisele S, Mwale A, Mwansa JK, Muma S, Chandwe M, Pilon R, Sandstrom P, Wu S, Yee K and Silverman MS, Efficacy of WHO recommendation for continued breastfeeding and maternal cART for prevention of perinatal and postnatal HIV transmission in Zambia, Journal of the International AIDS Society 2015, 18:19352, http://www.jiasociety.org/index.php/jias/article/view/19352

18. Gartland MG et al, Field effectiveness of combination antiretroviral prophylaxis for the prevention of mother-to-child HIV transmission in rural Zambia, AIDS 2013 May 15; 27(8): doi:10.1097/QAD.0b013e32835e3937, https://www.ncbi.nlm.nih.gov/pmc/articles/PMC3836017/pdf/nihms521144.pdf/

19. Luoga E et al, No HIV Transmission From Virally Suppressed Mothers During Breastfeeding in Rural Tanzania J Acquir Immune Defic Syndr 2018 Sep 1;79(1):e17-e20. doi: 10.1097/QAI.0000000000001758. https://pubmed.ncbi.nlm.nih.gov/29781882/ (accessed 6 Aug 2020)
20. Flynn PM et al, Association of Maternal Viral Load count with Perinatal HIV-1 Transmission Risk during Breastfeeding in the PROMISE Postpartum Component, poster presentation given at the International AIDS conference in Amsterdam July 2018 https://programme.aids2018.org/PAGMaterial/eposters/4897.pdf
21. Flynn PM et al for the PROMISE Study Team, Prevention of HIV-1 Transmission Through Breastfeeding: Efficacy and Safety of Maternal Antiretroviral Therapy Versus Infant Nevirapine Prophylaxis for Duration of Breastfeeding in HIV-1-Infected Women With High CD4 Cell Count (IMPAACT PROMISE): A Randomized, Open-Label, Clinical Trial. J Acquir Immune Defic Syndr 2018;77(4):383-392. doi: 10.1097/QAI.0000000000001612. https://www.ncbi.nlm.nih.gov/pubmed/29239901
22. Daniels B, Spooner E, Coutsoudis A. Getting to under 1% vertical HIV transmission: lessons from a breastfeeding cohort in South Africa, BMJ Global Health 2022;7:1-5, e009927. doi:10.1136/bmjgh-2022-009927. https://gh.bmj.com/content/7/9/e009927
23. Dunn DT, Newell ML, Ades AE, Peckham CS, Risk of human immunodeficiency virus type 1 transmission through breastfeeding. Lancet Sep 5, 1992;340:585-88. https://www.ncbi.nlm.nih.gov/pubmed/1355163
24. Nduati R, John G, Mbori-Ngacha D et al. Effect of breastfeeding and formula feeding on transmission of HIV-1: a randomized clinical trial. JAMA 2000;283(9):1167-74.
25. Coovadia HM, Rollins NC, Bland RM, Little K, Coutsoudis A, Bennish ML, Newell M-L. Mother-to-child transmission of HIV-1 infection during exclusive breastfeeding in the first 6 months of life: an intervention cohort study. Lancet 2007 March 31;369:1107-16. https://www.ncbi.nlm.nih.gov/pubmed/17398310
26. Kesho Bora Study Group, Triple antiretroviral compared with zidovudine and single-dose nevirapine prophylaxis during pregnancy and breastfeeding for prevention of mother-to-child transmission of HIV-1 (Kesho Bora study): a randomised controlled trial, Lancet 2011; DOI:10.1016/S1473-3099(10)70288-7 https://www.thelancet.com/journals/laninf/article/PIIS1473-3099
27. Nevrekar et al, Self-Reported Antiretroviral Adherence: Association with Maternal Viral Load Suppression in Postpartum Women Living with HIV-1 from Promoting Maternal and Infant Survival Everywhere (PROMISE), a Randomized Controlled Trial in Sub-Saharan Africa and India, JAIDS Journal of Acquired Immune Deficiency Syndromes: September 28, 2022 doi: 10.1097/QAI.0000000000003102 JAIDS 2022 https://journals.lww.com/jaids/Abstract/9900/Self_Reported_Antiretroviral_Adherence_.117.aspx
28. Nagot N et al and Philippe van de Perre, Extended pre-exposure prophylaxis with lopinavir-ritonavir versus lamivudine to prevent HIV-1 transmission through breastfeeding up to 50 weeks in infants in Africa (ANRS 12174): a randomised controlled trial Lancet 2016 Feb 6;387(10018):566-573. doi: 10.1016/S0140-6736(15)00984-8. Epub 2015 Nov 19 https://www.thelancet.

REFERENCES

com/journals/lancet/article/PIIS0140-6736(15)00984-8/fulltext
29. BHIVA guidelines for the management of HIV in pregnancy and postpartum 2018 (2020 third interim update) (See Section 9.4.4 Choosing to breastfeed in the UK. Pages 95-6) https://www.bhiva.org/file/5f1aab1ab9aba/BHIVA-Pregnancy-guidelines-2020-3rd-interim-update.pdf (accessed 30 Sept 2022)
30. Nashid N, Khan S, Loutfy M, et al. Breastfeeding by women living with human immunodeficiency virus in a resource-rich setting: a case series of maternal and infant management and outcomes. J Pediatric Infect Dis Soc. 2020;9(2):228-231. https://www.ncbi.nlm.nih.gov/pubmed/30753640
31. Garcia PM, Kalish LA, Pitt J, Minkoff H, Quinn TC, Burchett SK, Kornegay J, Jackson B, Moye J, Hanson C, Zorrilla C, Lew JF. Maternal levels of plasma human immunodeficiency virus type 1 RNA and the risk of perinatal transmission. Women and Infants Transmission Study Group. N Engl J Med. 1999 Aug 5;341(6):394-402. https://pubmed.ncbi.nlm.nih.gov/10432324/
32. UNAIDS 2016 The need for routine viral load testing. https://www.unaids.org/sites/default/files/media_asset/JC2845_en.pdf
33. Alcorn K, Viral Load Blips are important warning signals European study finds, AIDSMAP News, Oct 2022) https://www.aidsmap.com/news/oct-2022/low-level-hiv-and-viral-load-blips-are-important-warning-signals-european-study-finds#:~:text=already%20resistant%20virus.-,blip,a%20sign%20of%20virologic%20failure
34. Quinn TC et al. Viral load and heterosexual transmission of HIV type 1. Rakai Project Study Group. N Engl J Med 2000; 342: 921-929. http://www.nejm.org/doi/full/10.1056/NEJM200003303421303
35. The Swiss Statement http://www.aids.ch/e/fragen/pdf/swissguidelinesART.pdf
36. Vernazza P & Bernard EJ. HIV is not transmitted under fully suppressive therapy: The Swiss Statement – eight years later. Swiss Med Wkly. 2016;146:w14246, https://smw.ch/article/doi/smw.2016.14246
37. Rodger AJ, Sexual Activity Without Condoms and Risk of HIV Transmission in Serodifferent Couples When the HIV-Positive Partner Is Using Suppressive Antiretroviral Therapy JAMA. 2016;316(2):171-181. doi:10.1001/jama.2016.5148
38. Rodger AJ et al, Risk of HIV transmission through condomless sex in serodifferent gay couples with the HIV positive partner taking suppressive antiretroviral therapy (PARTNER): final results of a multicentre, prospective, observational study, https://doi.org/10.1016/S0140-6736(19)30418-0 Lancet 2019;393:2428-2438 published online 2 May 2019, print version 15 June 2019 https://www.thelancet.com/journals/lancet/article/PIIS0140-6736(19)30418-0/fulltext
39. Sibiude J et al, Update of perinatal human immunodeficiency virus type 1 transmission in France: zero transmission for 5482 mothers on continuous antiretroviral therapy from conception and with undetectable viral load at delivery, Clin Infect Dis 2023: 76(3):e590=e598. https://pubmed.ncbi.nlm.nih.gov/36037040/
40. Kahlert C, Aebi-Popp K, Bernasconi E, et al. Is breastfeeding an equipoise option in effectively treated HIV-infected mothers in a high-income setting? Swiss Medical Weekly. 2018 Jul 23;148:w14648. Available from: https://smw.ch/article/doi/smw.2018.14648

41. Vernazza, Interview by Eva Sommelatte, for Comite des Families, July 2021 https://www.comitedesfamilles.net/interview-du-professeur-pietro-vernazza-sur-le-theme-vih-et-allaitement/
42. ISOSS Report, 21 July 2021, https://www.gov.uk/government/publications/integrated-screening-outcomes-surveillance-service-isoss-annual-report/integrated-screening-outcomes-surveillance-service-isoss-annual-report-2021
43. ISOSS HIV Report October 2022 https://www.gov.uk/government/publications/infectious-diseases-in-pregnancy-screening-isoss-hiv-report-2022/isoss-hiv-report-2022#hiv-and-breastfeeding
44. Haberl L, Audebert F, Feiterna-Sperling C, et al. Not recommended, but done: breastfeeding with HIV in Germany. AIDS Patient Care STDS. 2021;35(2):33-38. https://www.ncbi.nlm.nih.gov/pubmed/33571048
45. Weiss F, von Both U, Rack-Hoch A, et al. Brief report: HIV-positive and breastfeeding in high-income settings: 5-year experience from a perinatal center in Germany. J Acquir Immune Defic Syndr. 2022;91(4):364-367. https://www.ncbi.nlm.nih.gov/pubmed/35944107
46. Crisinel PA, Kusejko K, Kahlert CR, Wagner N and Beyer LS. Successful implementation of new Swiss recommendations on breastfeeding of infants born to women living with HIV. European Journal of Obstetrics & Gynecology and Reproductive Biology, 2023;283:86–89 https://doi.org/10.1016/j.ejogrb.2023.02.013
47. Yusuf HE, Knott-Grasso MA, Anderson J, et al. Experience and outcomes of breastfed infants of women living with HIV in the United States: findings from a single-center breastfeeding support initiative. J Pediatric Infect Dis Soc. 2022;11(1):24-27. https://ncbi.nlm/nih.gov/pubmed/34888664
48. Koay WLA, Rakhmanina NY. Supporting mothers living with HIV in the United States who choose to breastfeed. J Pediatric Infect Dis Soc. 2022;11(5):239. https://www.ncbi.nlm.nih.gov/pubmed/35238385.
49. Abuogi L et al. Development and implementation of an interdisciplinary model for the management of breastfeeding in women with HIV in the United States: experience from the Children's Hospital Colorado Immunodeficiency Program, J Acquir Immune Defic Syndr 2023 online ahead of print Apr 27 https://pubmed.ncbi.nlm.nih.gov/37104739/
50. Tuthill EL, Tomori C, Van Natta M, Coleman JS. "In the United States, we say, 'no breastfeeding,' but that is no longer realistic": provider perspectives towards infant feeding among women living with HIV in the United States. J Int AIDS Soc. 2019;22(1):e25224. https://www.ncbi.nlm.nih/gov/pubmed/30657639
51. Prestileo T, Adriana S, Lorenza DM, Argo A. From undetectable equals untransmittable (U=U) to breastfeeding: is the jump short? Infect Dis Rep. 2022;14(2):220-227. https://www.ncbi.nlm.nih.gov/pubmed/35447879
52. Bansaccal N, HIV-Infected Mothers Who Decide to Breastfeed Their Infants Under Close Supervision in Belgium: About Two Cases, Front Pediatr 2020;8:248 https://www.frontiersin.org/articles/10.3389/fped.2020.00248/full
53. WHO-UNICEF 2016, Guideline: Updates on HIV and Infant Feeding, http://apps.who.int/iris/bitstream/10665/246260/1/9789241549707-eng.pdf

54. American Academy of Pediatrics, Infant Feeding and Transmission of Human Immunodeficiency Virus in the United States, Committee on Pediatric AIDS, Pediatrics, originally published online January 28, 2013, DOI: 10.1542/peds.2012-3543, Pediatrics 2013;131:391–396 available at http://pediatrics.aappublications.org/content/early/2013/01/23/peds.2012-3543
55. The Well Project, https://www.thewellproject.org/who-we-are/about-us
56. The US Panel on Treatment of HIV in Pregnancy and Prevention and Perinatal Transmission and the Panel on Antiretroviral Therapy and Medical Management of Children Living with HIV https://clinicalinfo.hiv.gov/en/guidelines/perinatal/infant-feeding-individuals-hiv-united-states?view=full
57. NAPWHA Breastfeeding for Women living with HIV in Australia, August 2021, https://napwha.org.au/wp-content/uploads/2021/08/NAPWHA-Living-Well-Breastfeeding-for-Women-living-with-HIV-Community-Resource-2021-web.pdf
58. New Zealand Ministry of Health, Pregnancy and breastfeeding with HIV, Nov 2020, https://www.health.govt.nz/your-health/conditions-and-treatments/diseases-and-illnesses/hiv-aids/pregnancy-and-breastfeeding-hiv#

Chapter 3: Enlisting help and advance planning

1. BHIVA guidelines for the management of HIV in pregnancy and postpartum 2018 (2020 third interim update) (See Section 9.4.4 Choosing to breastfeed in the UK. Pages 95-6) https://www.bhiva.org/file/5f1aab1ab9aba/BHIVA-Pregnancy-guidelines-2020-3rd-interim-update.pdf (accessed 30 Sept 2022)
2. The US Panel on Treatment of HIV in Pregnancy and Prevention and Perinatal Transmission and the Panel on Antiretroviral Therapy and Medical Management of Children Living with HIV https://clinicalinfo.hiv.gov/en/guidelines/perinatal/infant-feeding-individuals-hiv-united-states?view=full
3. ISOSS, UCL Great Ormond Street Institute of Child Health, 30 Guilford Street, London WC1N 1EH. Email: isoss@ucl.ac.uk website at https://www.isoss-online.org
4. ISOSS Annual Report, July 2021, https://www.gov.uk/government/publications/integrated-screening-outcomes-surveillance-service-isoss-annual-report/integrated-screening-outcomes-surveillance-service-isoss-annual-report-2021
5. Dr Shema Tariq, NOURISH Webinar, October 2022
6. Van de Perre P, Kankasa C, Nagot N, et al. Pre-exposure prophylaxis for infants exposed to HIV through breast feeding. BMJ. 2017;356:j1053. https://pubmed.ncbi.nlm.nih.gov/28279960/
7. BHIVA Statement on Covid, 25 March 2020, (British lockdown commenced 23 March 2020) https://www.bhiva.org/management-of-a-woman-living-with-HIV-while-pregnant-during-Coronavirus-COVID-19 (accessed 1 September 2021).
8. Who's Who in Lactation in UK, https://www.lcgb.org/wp-content/uploads/2018/02/Whos-Who-2017-Oct-17-1.pdf
9. Lactation Consultants of Great Britain, Find a Lactation Consultant close to your Postcode, see https://lcgb.org/find-an-ibclc/
10. National Breastfeeding Helpline, run by volunteer breastfeeding supporters

from the main breastfeeding groups, telephone 0300 100 0212 from 9.30am to 9.30pm every day
11. https://gpifn.org.uk/uk-infant-feeding-support/
12. https://www.nhs.uk/service-search/other-services/Breastfeeding-support-services/LocationSearch/360
13. Sarah Oakley, Choosing a breast pump. https://sarahoakleylactation.co.uk/choosing-a-breast-pump/
14. Stuart-Macadam P and Dettwyler KA. Breastfeeding: Biocultural Perspectives, ISBN 0-202-01192-5, Aldine de Gruyter, New York, 1995.
15. Personal communication with a client

Chapter 4: The transformational effect of ART, and ART + EBF

1. CHIVA Standards of Care for Infants, Children, and Young People with HIV (Including infants born to mothers with HIV) 2017, https://www.chiva.org.uk/files/5215/3987/5455/CHIVA_STANDARDS_2017.pdf
2. WHO 2009, HIV and infant feeding, Revised Principles and Recommendations. Rapid Advice, November 2009. Available at http://whqlibdoc.who.int/publications/2009/9789241598873_eng.pdf
3. Newell M-L et al. Mortality of Infected and Uninfected Infants Born to HIV-infected Mothers in Africa: A pooled analysis, Lancet 2004; 364: 1236–43
4. CDC Recommendations of the U.S. Public Health Service Task Force on the Use of Zidovudine to Reduce Perinatal Transmission of Human Immunodeficiency Virus. MMWR 1994;43 (no. RR-11). https://www.cdc.gov/mmwr/preview/mmwrhtml/00032271.htm
5. Mofensen L. Short-course zidovudine for prevention of perinatal infection, Lancet 1998;353(9155):766-767 https://www.thelancet.com/journals/lancet/article/PIIS0140-6736(99)90028-4/fulltext
6. Chibwesha CJ, Giganti MJ, Putta N, Chintu N, Mulindwa J, Dorton BJ, Chi BH, Stringer JS, Stringer EM. Optimal Time on HAART for Prevention of Mother-to-Child Transmission of HIV. J Acquir Immune Defic Syndr. 2011 Oct 1;58(2):224-8. doi: 10.1097/QAI.0b013e318229147e, http://www.ncbi.nlm.nih.gov/pubmed/21709566 Full-text free access https://www.ncbi.nlm.nih.gov/pmc/articles/PMC3605973/pdf/nihms437123.pdf
7. Dr Shema Tariq, NOURISH webinar, October 2022
8. BHIVA guidelines for the management of HIV in pregnancy and postpartum 2018 (2020 third interim update) https://www.bhiva.org/file/5f1aab1ab9aba/BHIVA-Pregnancy-guidelines-2020-3rd-interim-update.pdf
9. UNAIDS1998, HIV and infant feeding, a Review of Transmission though Breastfeeding, p 12 https://www.unaids.org/sites/default/files/media_asset/jc180-hiv-infantfeeding-3_en_0.pdf (accessed 25 June 2023)
10. Dr Deborah Cohan, Dept of Obstetrics Gynecology and Reproductive Sciences, University of California, San Francisco, personal communication
11. Recommendations for the Use of Antiretroviral Drugs during Pregnancy and Interventions to Reduce Perinatal HIV Transmission in the United States, Guidelines for the Use of Antiretroviral Agents in Pediatric Infection, section on ARV prophylaxis for Newborns at low risk of Perinatal HIV transmission who are Breastfed at https://clinicalinfo.hiv.gov/en/guidelines/perinatal/

management-infants-arv-hiv-exposure-infection?view=full
12. Nashid N, Khan S, Loutfy M, et al. Breastfeeding by women living with human immunodeficiency virus in a resource-rich setting: a case series of maternal and infant management and outcomes. J Pediatric Infect Dis Soc. 2020;9(2):228-231. https://www.ncbi.nlm.nih.gov/pubmed/30753640
13. Lees EA, Tickner N, Lyall H et al, Infant postnatal prophylaxis following maternal viraemia during breastfeeding. AIDS 2023;37(7):1185-1186 https://pubmed.ncbi.nlm.nih.gov/37139658/

Chapter 5: Why exclusive breastfeeding matters

1. WHO Expert Consultation that completed the systematic review of the optimal duration of exclusive breastfeeding, A54/INF.DOC./4). See also resolution WHA54.2. (Geneva, 28–30 March 2001)
2. Duitjes L et al, Prolonged and Exclusive Breastfeeding Reduces the Risk of Infectious Diseases in Infancy, Pediatrics 2010 Jul;126(1):e18-25. doi: 10.1542/peds.2008-3256. Epub 2010 Jun 21. https://pubmed.ncbi.nlm.nih.gov/20566605/
3. Kramer MS, Kakuma R. The optimal duration of exclusive breastfeeding: A systematic review. Adv Exp Med Biol 2004, 554:63-77
4. American Academy of Pediatrics, Policy Statement: Breastfeeding and the Use of Human Milk, 27 June 2022. Pediatrics. 2022;150(1):e2022057988 https://publications.aap.org/pediatrics/article/150/1/e2022057988/188347/Policy-Statement-Breastfeeding-and-the-Use-of?s
5. UNICEF, Breastfeeding in the UK, https://www.unicef.org.uk/babyfriendly/about/breastfeeding-in-the-uk/
6. WHO Fact sheet on breastfeeding, https://www.who.int/en/news-room/fact-sheets/detail/infant-and-young-child-feeding
7. De Onis et al, WHO Growth standards for infants and young children, Arch Pediatr. 2009 Jan;16(1):47-53. doi: 10.1016/j.arcped.2008.10.010. Epub 2008 Nov 25. http://www.ncbi.nlm.nih.gov/pubmed/19036567
8. Brown K et al. Infant feeding practices and their relationship with diarrhoeal and other diseases in Huascar (Lima) Peru. Pediatrics, 1989, 83:31–40.
9. Almroth S, Bidinger PD. No need for water supplementation for exclusively breast-fed infants under hot and arid conditions, Transactions of The Royal Society of Tropical Medicine and Hygiene 1990;84(4):602-604, 1 Aug 1990 https://doi.org/10.1016/0035-9203(90)90056-K
10. Edney JM, Kovats S, Filippi V and Nakstad B (2022) A systematic review of hot weather impacts on infant feeding practices in low-and middle-income countries. Front. Pediatr. 10:930348. doi: 10.3389/fped.2022.930348
11. WHO 2001 The optimal duration of exclusive breastfeeding. Report of an expert consultation. Geneva, WHO (WHO/NHD/01.09, WHO/FCH/CAH/01.24) March 2001.
12. WHO 2009 Model Chapter on Infant and Young Child Feeding, Model Chapter for textbooks http://whqlibdoc.who.int/publications/2009/9789241597494_eng.pdf
13. Coutsoudis A, Pillay K, Spooner E, Kuhn L, Coovadia HM. Influence of infant-feeding patterns on early mother-to-child transmission of HIV-1 in Durban, South Africa: a prospective cohort study. South African Vitamin A

Study Group. Lancet. 1999 Aug 7;354(9177):471-6.
14. Coutsoudis A, Pillay K, Kuhn L, Spooner E, Tsai W-Y, Coovadia HM for the South African Vitamin A Study Group. Method of feeding and transmission of HIV-1 from mothers to children by 15 months of age: prospective cohort study from Durban, South Africa. AIDS 2001;15:379-387
15. Iliff PJ, Piwoz EG, Tavengwa NV, Zunguza CD, Marinda ET, Nathoo KJ, Moulton LH, Ward BJ, the ZVITAMBO study group and Humphrey JH. Early exclusive breastfeeding reduces the risk of postnatal HIV-1 transmission and increases HIV-free survival. AIDS 2005, 19:699–708
16. Coovadia HM, Rollins NC, Bland RM, Little K, Coutsoudis A, Bennish ML, Newell M-L. Mother-to-child transmission of HIV-1 infection during exclusive breastfeeding in the first 6 months of life: an intervention cohort study. Lancet 2007 March 31;369:1107-16.
17. Smith MM and Kuhn L, Exclusive breast-feeding: does it have the potential to reduce breast-feeding transmission of HIV-1?. Nutrition Reviews 2000;58(11):333-340.
18. Lunney KM, Iliff P, Mutasa K, Ntozini R, Magder LS, Moulton LH and Humphrey JH. Associations between Breast Milk Viral Load, Mastitis, Exclusive Breast-Feeding, and Postnatal Transmission of HIV Clinical Infectious Diseases 2010; 50:762–769
19. Kuhn L, Sinkala M, Semrau K, Kankasa C, Kasonde P, Mwiya M, Hu C-C, Tsai W-Y, Thea D and Aldrovandi GM. Elevations in Mortality Associated with Weaning Persist into the Second Year of Life among Uninfected Children Born to HIV-Infected Mothers. Clin Infect Dis. 2010;50:437-444.
20. Catassi C, Bonucci A, Coppa GV et al. Intestinal permeability changes during the first month: effect of natural versus artificial feeding. J Pedatr Gastroenterol Nutr 1995;21:383-6.
21. Filteau SM, Rollins NC, Coutsoudis A, Sullivan KR, Willumsen JF, Tomkins AM. The effect of antenatal vitamin A and beta-carotene supplementation on gut integrity of infants of HIV-infected South African women. J Pediatr Gastroenterol Nutr. 2001 Apr;32(4):464-70.
22. Smith A and Heads J, Breast Pathology, in Walker M (Ed) Core curriculum for lactation consultant practice, 2002. Jones & Bartlett Inc and International Lactation Consultant Association.
23. Lawrence RA and Lawrence RM, 1999, Breastfeeding: a guide for the medical profession, 5th ed, Mosby Inc, St Louis, Missouri.
24. Amir L, Hoover K, Mulford C. Candidiasis & Breastfeeding, Lactation Consultant Series Unit 18, La Leche League International 1995.
25. Lake AM. Dietary protein enterocolitis. Curr Allergy Rep. 2001 Jan;1(1):76-9.
26. Fetherston C. Mastitis in lactating women: physiology or pathology? Breastfeed Rev 2001 Mar;9(1):5-12.
27. Cox DB, Kent JC, Casey TM, Owens RA, Hartmann PE. Breast growth and the urinary excretion of lactose during human pregnancy and early lactation: endocrine relationships. Exp Physiol 1999;84:421-34.
28. Stelwagen K, Farr VC, McFadden HA, Prosser CG, Davis SR. Time course of milk accumulation – induced opening of the mammary tight junctions and blood clearance of milk components. Am J Physiol Regul Integr Comp Physiol 1997;273:R379-86.
29. Hartmann PE, Kulski JK. Changes in the composition of the mammary

REFERENCES

secretion of women after abrupt termination of breast feeding. J Physiol. 1978 Feb;275:1-11.
30. Kuhn L, Sinkala M, Kankasa C, Semrau K, Kasonde P, Scott N, Mwiya M, Cheswa V, Walter J, Wei-Yann T, Aldrovandi GM, and Thea DM. High Uptake of Exclusive Breastfeeding and Reduced Early Post-Natal HIV Transmission. PLoS ONE Dec 2007; 2(12): e1363. doi:10.1371/journal.pone.

Chapter 6: Beginning breastfeeding, positioning and attachment, latching techniques

1. McAndrew F, Thompson J, Fellows L, Large A, Speed M and Renfrew MJ, Infant Feeding Survey 2010, Health and Social Care Information Centre https://files.digital.nhs.uk/publicationimport/pub08xxx/pub08694/ifs-uk-2010-sum.pdf
2. NCT, Labour pain relief, https://www.nct.org.uk/labour-birth/your-pain-relief-options/labour-pain-relief-intramuscular-opioids-pethidine-and-diamorphine#:~:text=Pethidine%2C%20diamorphine%20and%20other%20opioids,Hemati%20et%20al%2C%202018).
3. BPNI Maharashtra, Breast Crawl video, https://bpnimaharashtra.org/wp-content/uploads/2019/11/2_English-Breast-Crawl-Video-Script-_-FAQ.pdf
4. Maher, SM. An overview of solutions to breastfeeding and sucking problems, La Leche League International, publication No.67 of October 1988.
5. Breastfeeding.Support, Breastfeeding Positions for Newborns, https://breastfeeding.support/breastfeeding-positions-for-newborns/
6. La Leche League, Positioning & Attachment, https://www.laleche.org.uk/positioning-attachment/ and https://www.llli.org/breastfeeding-info/positioning/
7. Global Health Media videos https://globalhealthmedia.org/videos/
8. Suzanne Colson, Biological Nurturing, http://www.biologicalnurturing.com/pages/message.html
9. Milinco M, Travan L, Cattaneo, A. et al. Effectiveness of biological nurturing on early breastfeeding problems: a randomized controlled trial. Int Breastfeed J 15, 21 (2020). https://doi.org/10.1186/s13006-020-00261-4 , https://internationalbreastfeedingjournal.biomedcentral.com/articles/10.1186/
10. UNICEF Baby Friendly Refresher Sheet 3, https://www.unicef.org.uk/babyfriendly/wp-content/uploads/sites/2/2020/04/Unicef-UK-Baby-Friendly-Initiative-education-refresher-sheet-3.pdf
11. IABLE latching videos https://www.youtube.com/watch?v=0I-OAr7Dr48
12. Global Health Media, Attaching your baby to the breast, https://globalhealthmedia.org/videos/attaching-your-baby-at-the-breast/
13. Virginia Thorley, personal communication

Chapter 7: Lactation management for mothers

1. Morrison P, How Often does breastfeeding really fail?, Breastfeeding Today, 19 February 2016, https://www.llli.org/how-often-does-breastfeeding-really-fail/
2. International Lactation Consultant Association 2013; Core Curriculum for Lactation Consultant Practice, Part 3, Anatomy & Physiology, Jones & Bartlett Learning publishers, Massachusetts

3. Dr Jack Newman on swallowing, https://www.youtube.com/watch?v=7giyNvlCW18
4. Minchin MK, author of Breastfeeding Matters: what we need to know about infant feeding (Alma Publications, 4th edition) generously provided comments and input to this section on milk transfer, suckling and swallowing.
5. Woolridge MW, Fisher C. Colic, "overfeeding", and symptoms of lactose malabsorption in the breast-fed baby: a possible artifact of feed management? Lancet. 1988;2(8607):382-4. https://pubmed.ncbi.nlm.nih.gov/2899785/
6. Cox DB, Kent JC, Casey TM, Owens RA, Hartmann PE. Breast growth and the urinary excretion of lactose during human pregnancy and early lactation: endocrine relationships. Exp Physiol 1999;84:421-34.
7. Stelwagen K, Farr VC, McFadden HA, Prosser CG, Davis SR. Time course of milk accumulation – induced opening of the mammary tight junctions and blood clearance of milk components. Am J Physiol Regul Integr Comp Physiol 1997;273:R379-86.
8. Kuhn L, Sinkala M, Kankasa C, Semrau K, Kasonde P, Scott N, Mwiya M, Cheswa V, Walter J, Wei-Yann T, Aldrovandi GM, and Thea DM. High Uptake of Exclusive Breastfeeding and Reduced Early Post-Natal HIV Transmission. PLoS ONE Dec 2007; 2(12): e1363. doi:10.1371/journal.pone.0001363
9. Walker M, (Engorgement, p 501), Breastfeeding Management for the Clinician, Using the Evidence, Jones & Bartlett Learning, Publishers, Massachusetts, 2014
10. Desmarais L and Browne S, Inadequate weight gain in breastfeeding infants; assessments and resolutions. Lactation Consultant Series Unit 8, La Leche League International.
11. Perlman NC & Carussi DA. Retained Placenta after Vaginal Delivery, risk factors and management, Int J Women's Health 2019. https://www.ncbi.nlm.nih.gov/pmc/articles/PMC6789409/#:~:text=If%20the%20placenta%20or%20pieces,management%20with%20dilation%20and%20curettage
12. GP Infant Feeding Network, Anatomy & Physiology https://gpifn.org.uk/anatomy-and-physiology/
13. Kent J et al, Longitudinal changes in breastfeeding patterns from 1 to 6 months of lactation. Breastfeed Med 2013;8(4):401-7. doi: 10.1089/bfm.2012.0141. Epub 2013 Apr 5. https://pubmed.ncbi.nlm.nih.gov/23560450/
14. World Health Organization Child Growth Standards, https://www.who.int/tools/child-growth-standards/standards/weight-for-age

Chapter 8: Mixed breastfeeding after six months

1. Goldman, AS, Modulation of the Gastrointestinal Tract of Infants by Human Milk. Interfaces and Interactions. An Evolutionary Perspective, The Journal of Nutrition 2000;130(2):426S–431S, https://doi.org/10.1093/jn/130.2.426S https://academic.oup.com/jn/article/130/2/426S/4686444
2. Ngoma M, Raha A, Elong A, Pilon R, Mwansa J, Mutale W, Yee K, Chisele S,

REFERENCES

Wu S, Chandawe M, Mumba S and Silverman MS (citation) Interim Results of HIV Transmission Rates Using a Lopinavir/ritonavir based regimen and the New WHO Breast Feeding Guidelines for PMTCT of HIV International Congress of Antimicrobial Agents and Chemotherapy (ICAAC) Chicago Il, Sep19,2011. H1-1153, available at http://www.icaac.org/index.php/component/content/article/9-newsroom/169-preliminary-results-of-hiv-transmission-rates-using-a-lopinavirritonavir-lpvr-aluvia-based-regimen-and-the-new-who-breast-feeding-guidelines-for-pmtct-of-hiv-

3. M Silverman, personal communication, 2 Oct 2011
4. Sint TT, Lovich R, Hammond W, Kim M, Melillo S, Lu L, Ching P, Marcy J, Rollins N, Koumans EH, Heap AN, Brewinski-Isaacs M; Child Survival Working Group of the Interagency Task Team on the Prevention and Treatment of HIV infection in Pregnant Women, Mothers and Children. Challenges in infant and young child nutrition in the context of HIV. AIDS. 2013 Nov;27 Suppl 2:S169-77. doi: 10.1097/QAD.0000000000000089. http://www.ncbi.nlm.nih.gov/pubmed/24361626
5. BHIVA guidelines for the management of HIV in pregnancy and postpartum 2018 (2020 third interim update) https://www.bhiva.org/pregnancy-guidelines (accessed 28 October 2022)
6. WHO-UNICEF 2016, Guideline: Updates on HIV and Infant Feeding, http://apps.who.int/iris/bitstream/10665/246260/1/9789241549707-eng.pdf
7. WHO Complementary Feeding, http://www.who.int/nutrition/topics/complementary_feeding/en/
8. Morrison P, HIV and breastfeeding: the untold story, Chapter 6, February 2022, Pinter & Martin, London
9. Victora CG et al, Association between breastfeeding and intelligence, educational attainment, and income at 30 years of age: a prospective birth cohort study from Brazil, Lancet 2015;3(4);e199-e205, https://www.thelancet.com/journals/langlo/article/PIIS2214-109X(15)70002-1/abstract)
10. Goldman, A.; Goldblum, R.; Garza, C., Immunologic components in human milk during the second year of lactation. Acta Paediatrica 1983, 72, (3), 461-462.
11. Bradley J; Baldwin S; Armstrong H. Breastfeeding: a neglected household-level weaning-food resource. In: UNICEF 1987 with SIDA and International Development Research Centre, Canada. Improving young child feeding in eastern and southern Africa. Household-level food technology. Proceedings of a workshop held in Nairobi, Kenya, 12-16 October 1987, edited by D. Alnwick, S. Moses and O.G. Schmidt. Ottawa, Canada, International Development Research Centre, 1988. 7-33. (IDRC-265e). Full-text of workshop available at http://idl-bnc.idrc.ca/dspace/bitstream/10625/17651/1/28523_p7-33.pdf
12. Frongillo EA, Habicht J-P, Investigating the weanling's dilemma: lessons from Honduras. Nutr Rev 1997;55:390-395. https://pubmed.ncbi.nlm.nih.gov/9420449/
13. Prameela KK & Mohamed AEK. Breast Milk Immunoprotection and the Common Mucosal Immune System: a Review, Mal J Nutr 16(1): 1 - 11, 2010, available at http://nutriweb.org.my/publications/mjn0016/Mhmd-Breastmik(edSP)1-11.pdf

14. La Leche League International, Breastfeeding Beyond a Year, Best Beginnings, https://www.laleche.org.uk/breastfeeding-beyond-a-year/
15. Piwoz EG, Huffman SL, Lusk D, Zehner ER, O'Gara C, Issues, Risks, and Challenges of Early Breastfeeding Cessation to Reduce Postnatal Transmission of HIV in Africa, For the Support for Analysis and Research in Africa (SARA) Project, Operated by the Academy for Educational Development, 2001. https://pdfs.semanticscholar.org/da62/aa8ffd13b771c34ca4c6b72400c9bf379a67.pdf
16. ISOSS Annual Report: https://www.gov.uk/government/publications/integrated-screening-outcomes-surveillance-service-isoss-annual-report/integrated-screening-outcomes-surveillance-service-isoss-annual-report-2021
17. Minchin M, Milk Matters: infant feeding & immune disorder, publisher Milk Matters Pty Ltd. Melbourne, 2015, ISBN 978095318319 Free download of book, https://infantfeedingmatters.com/milk-matters/
18. Amy Brown, Baby-led weaning: the evidence to date, Curr Nutr Rep 2017, DOI 10.1007/s13668-017-0201-2 at https://link.springer.com/article/10.1007/s13668-017-0201-2
19. Maritz ER, Kidd M, Cotton MF, Premasticating food for weaning African infants: a possible vehicle for transmission of HIV. Pediatrics 2011 Sep;128(3):e579-90. doi: 10.1542/peds.2010-3109. Epub 2011 Aug 28. https://www.ncbi.nlm.nih.gov/pubmed/21873699

Chapter 9: Weaning from the breast

1. WHO-UNICEF 2016, Guideline: Updates on HIV and Infant Feeding, http://apps.who.int/iris/bitstream/10665/246260/1/9789241549707-eng.pdf
2. La Leche League International, How do I wean my baby? https://www.llli.org/breastfeeding-info/weaning-how-to/
3. NHS, Your baby's first solid foods, https://www.nhs.uk/conditions/baby/weaning-and-feeding/babys-first-solid-foods/
4. Tette EMA et al, Feeding practices and malnutrition at the Princess Marie Louise Children's Hospital, Accra: what has changed after 80 years? BMC Nutrition 2016;2:42. https://bmcnutr.biomedcentral.com/articles/10.1186/s40795-016-0082-6
5. Piwoz EG, Huffman SL, Lusk D, Zehner ER, O'Gara C, Issues, Risks, and Challenges of Early Breastfeeding Cessation to Reduce Postnatal Transmission of HIV in Africa, For the Support for Analysis and Research in Africa (SARA) Project, Operated by the Academy for Educational Development, 2001
6. Breastfeeding.support, Can you get pregnant while breastfeeding? 13 Nov 2019, https://breastfeeding.support/can-you-get-pregnant-while-breastfeeding/
7. Brown A, Why breastfeeding grief and trauma matter, 2022, Pinter & Martin, London
8. Kuhn L, Kim H-Y, Walter J, Thea DM, Sinkala M, Mwiya M, Kankasa C, Decker D, Aldrovandi GM, HIV-1 Concentrations in Human Breast Milk Before and After Weaning, Sci Transl Med, Vol. 5, Issue 181, p. 181ra51, Sci. Transl. Med. DOI: 10.1126/scitranslmed.3005113, Apr 2013 http://stm.

sciencemag.org/content/5/181/181ra51.full.html
9. ILCA, Core Curriculum for Lactation Consultant Practice, third Edition, 2013, Jones & Bartlett publishers, Massachusetts, USA)

Chapter 10: Expressing, pumping, storing breastmilk, and breastmilk-feeding

1. WHO 2001. The optimal duration of exclusive breastfeeding. Report of an expert consultation. Geneva, WHO (WHO/NH D/01.09, WHO/FCH/CAH/01.24) March 2001.
2. Academy of Breastfeeding Medicine, Clinical Protocol #8: Human Milk Storage, Information for Home Use for Full-Term Infants (Original Protocol March 2004, 2010, Revised 2017 https://abm.memberclicks.net/assets/DOCUMENTS/PROTOCOLS/8-human-milk-storage-protocol-english.pdf
3. Brusseau R 1998, Analysis of refrigerated human milk following infant feeding (unpublished study).
4. Read JS, Non-antiretroviral Approaches to Prevention of Breast Milk Transmission of HIV-1: Exclusive Breastfeeding, Early Weaning, Treatment of Expressed Breast Milk, Chapter 14, A.P. Kourtis and M. Bulterys (eds.), Human Immunodeficiency Virus type 1 (HIV-1) and Breastfeeding, Advances in Experimental Medicine and Biology 743, DOI 10.1007/978-1-4614-2251-8_14, © Springer Science+Business Media, LLC 2012
5. Stanford University https://med.stanford.edu/newborns/professional-education/breastfeeding/hand-expressing-milk.html
6. Global Health Media, how to express breastmilk, https://globalhealthmedia.org/portfolio-items/how-to-express-breastmilk/
7. WHO 2000, HIV & Infant feeding counselling: a training course, a trainer's guide WHO/FCH/CAH/00.3
8. Breastfeeding.Support on cup-feeding, https://breastfeeding.support/cup-feeding-newborn/
9. LA Lactation LLC Video on cupfeeding https://www.youtube.com/watch?v=X2t57eNGMEs
10. Cup-feeding prem baby video https://www.facebook.com/mybabyexperts/videos/830730858286919
11. Global Health Media, cup-feeding https://www.youtube.com/watch?v=-6AU6y6qatc
12. Minnesota WIC, paced bottle-feeding https://www.health.state.mn.us/docs/people/wic/localagency/wedupdate/moyr/2017/topic/1115feeding.pdf
13. La Leche League UK https://www.laleche.org.uk/nursing-supplementers/
14. NHS video. https://www.youtube.com/watch?v=d4KQULz9u5Q

Chapter 11: Pasteurising/flash-heating

1. BHIVA, HIV and breastfeeding your baby, Safer Triangle booklet (Leaflet 1) https://www.bhiva.org/file/5bfd3080d2027/BF-Leaflet-1.pdf
2. Orloff SL, Wallingford JC, McDougal JS 1993, Inactivation of human immunodeficiency virus type 1 in human milk: effects of intrinsic factors in human milk and of pasteurization. J Hum Lact 9(1):13-17.
3. Chantry CJ, Morrison P, Panchula J, Rivera C, Hillyer G, Zorilla C, Diaz C. Effects of lipolysis or heat treatment on HIV-1 provirus in breast milk.. J

Acquir Immune Defic Syndr 2000;24(4):325-9.
4. Jeffery BS, Mercer KG, Pretoria pasteurisation: a potential method for the reduction of postnatal mother to child transmission of the human immunodeficiency virus, J Trop Pediatr 2000;46(4):219-23.
5. Jeffery BS, Webber L, Mokhondo KR and Erasmus D, Determination of the Effectiveness of Inactivation of Human Immunodeficiency Virus by Pretoria Pasteurization, J Trop Pediatr 2001; 47(6):345-349.
6. Jeffery BS, Soma-Pillay P, Makin J and Mooman G, The effect of Pretoria pasteurization on bacterial contamination of hand-expressed human breastmilk. J Trop Pediatr 2004;49(4):240-244.
7. Israel-Ballard K, Chantry C, Dewey K et al. Viral, nutritional and bacterial safety of flash-heated and Pretoria pasteurized beast milk to prevent mother-to-child transmission of HIV in resource-poor countries: a pilot study. J Acquir Immune Defic Syndr. 2005;40:175-181.
8. Israel-Ballard K, Flash-heated and Pretoria Pasteurized destroys HIV in breast milk & Preserves Nutrients!, Advanced Biotech Sept 2008, http://www.advancedbiotech.in/51%20Flash%20heated.pdf
9. Israel-Ballard K, Donovan R, Chantry C, Coutsoudis A, Sheppard H, Sibeko L and Abrams B. Flash heat inactivation of HIV-1 in human milk. A potential method to reduce postnatal transmission in developing countries. J Acquir Immun Defic Syndr 45 (3): 318-323, May 2007
10. Volk ML, Hanson CV, Israel-Ballard K, Chantry CJ, Inactivation of Cell-Associated and Cell-Free HIV-1 by Flash-Heat Treatment of Breast Milk. J Acquir Immune Defic Syndr 2010;53(5):665-666.
11. Israel-Ballard KA et al. Vitamin content of breast milk from HIV-1–infected mothers before and after flash-heat treatment. J Acquir Immune Defic Syndr 2008;48: 444–449.
12. Hoque SA, Hoshino H, Anwar KS, Tanaka A, Shinagawa M, Hayakawa Y, Okitsu S, Wada Y, Ushijima H. Transient heating of expressed breast milk up to 65°C inactivates HIV-1 in milk: a simple, rapid, and cost-effective method to prevent postnatal transmission. J Med Virol. 2013 Feb;85(2):187-93. doi: 10.1002/jmv.23457. Epub 2012 Nov 21. http://www.ncbi.nlm.nih.gov/pubmed/23172701
13. Israel-Ballard K, Coutsoudis A, Chantry CJ, Sturm AW, Karim F, Sibeko L, Abrams B. Bacterial safety of flash-heated and unheated expressed breastmilk during storage. J Trop Pediatr. 2006;52:399–405.
14. Chantry CJ, Weideman J, Buehring G, Peerson JM, Hayfron K, K'Aluoch O, Lonnerdal B, Israel-Ballard K, Coutsoudis A and Abrams B. Effect of Flash-Heat Treatment on Antimicrobial Activity of Breastmilk Breastfeeding Medicine 2011;6(3):111-116, DOI: 10.1089/bfm.2010.0078
15. Chantry CJ, Israel-Ballard K, Moldoveanu Z, Peerson J, Coutsoudis, Sibeko L and Abrams B. Effect of Flash-heat Treatment on Immunoglobulins in Breastmilk. J Acquir Immune Defic Syndr. 2009 July 1; 51(3): 264–267. doi:10.1097/QAI.0b013e3181aa12f2. available at http://www.ncbi.nlm.nih.gov/pmc/articles/PMC2779733/pdf/nihms126967.pdf (accessed 5 December 2010)
16. Zimbabwe Ministry of Health and Child Welfare, Infant Feeding and HIV/AIDS; guidelines for health workers in Zimbabwe; June 12, 2000.
17. Reimers P, personal communication in GOLD10 Forum, www.goldconf.com

May 2010
18. Chantry CJ, Young SL, Rennie W, Ngonyani M, Mashi C, Israel-Ballard K, Peerson J, Nyambo MD, Matee M, Ash D, Dewey K and Koniz-Booher P. Feasibility of Using Flash-heated Breastmilk as an Infant Feeding Option for HIV-exposed, Uninfected Infants after 6 Months of Age in Urban Tanzania Journal of Acquired Immune Deficiency Syndromes 2012, DOI: 10.1097/QAI.0b013e31824fc06e
19. Mbuya MNN, Humphrey JH, Majo F, Chasekwa B, Jenkins A, Israel-Ballard K, Muti M, Paul KH, Madzima RC, Moulton LH and Stoltzfus RJ. Heat treatment of expressed breast milk is a feasible option for feeding HIV-exposed, uninfected children after 6 months of age in rural Zimbabwe. J Nutr 2010, Epub ahead of print June 23, 2010 as doi: 10.3945/jn.110.122457
20. TenHam WH. Heat treatment of expressed breast milk as in-home procedure to limit mother-to-child transmission of HIV: A systematic review. Submitted to School of Nursing Science, North-West University, Potchefstroom, South Africa November 2009 available at http://dspace.nwu.ac.za/bitstream/10394/3745/1/TenHam_HW.pdf
21. Read JS, Non-antiretroviral Approaches to Prevention of Breast Milk Transmission of HIV-1: Exclusive Breastfeeding, Early Weaning, Treatment of Expressed Breast Milk, Chapter 14, A.P. Kourtis and M. Bulterys (eds.), Human Immunodeficiency Virus type 1 (HIV-1) and Breastfeeding, Advances in Experimental Medicine and Biology 743, DOI 10.1007/978-1-4614-2251-8_14, © Springer Science+Business Media, LLC 2012
22. Minchin M. Milk Matters: Infant Feeding and Immune Disorder, available at https://infantfeedingmatters.com/
23. UC Berkeley News Press Release 2007, https://newsarchive.berkeley.edu/news/media/releases/2007/05/21_breastmilk.shtml
24. Mother's Milk Bank, North East, Storing, Defrosting, and Warming Pasteurized Donor Human Milk, https://milkbankne.org/wp-content/uploads/2021/06/Storing-and-Thawing-Donor-Milk-1.pdf

Chapter 12: Breast problems

1. Piwoz E & Ross J, HIV and Infant Feeding, Knowledge Gaps and challenges for the future, Joint WABA/UNICEF HIV colloquium, Arusha, Tanzania 2002
2. Desmarais L & Browne S. Inadequate weight gain in breastfeeding infants; assessments and resolutions, Lactation consultant Series Unit 8, La Leche League International; 1990.
3. WHO 2000, Mastitis, http://apps.who.int/iris/bitstream/handle/10665/66230/WHO_FCH_CAH_00.13_eng.pdf
4. Riordan J, Nichols F. A descriptive study of lactation mastitis in long-term breastfeeding women. J Hum Lact 1990;6:53-58.
5. Kinlay JR, O'Connell DL, Kinlay S. Incidence of mastitis in breastfeeding women during the first six months after delivery: a prospective cohort study. Med J Aust 1998:310-12
6. Willumsen JF, Filteau SM, Coutsoudis A, Uebel KE, Newell ML, Tomkins AM. Subclinical mastitis as a risk factor for mother-infant HIV transmission. Adv Exp Med Biol. 2000;478:211-23.

7. Willumsen JF, Filteau SM, Coutsoudis A, Newell ML, Rollins NC, Coovadia HM, Tomkins AM, Breastmilk RNA viral load in HIV-infected South African women: effects of subclinical mastitis and infant feeding. AIDS. 2003 Feb 14;17(3):407-14.
8. Embree JE, Njenga S, Datta P, Nagelkerke NJD, Ndinya-Achola JO, Mohammed Z, Ramdahin S, Bwayo JJ, Plummer F, Risk factors for postnatal mother-child transmission of HIV, AIDS 2000, 14:2535-2541.

Chapter 13: Nipple problems

1. La Leche League Great Britain, nipple pain, https://www.laleche.org.uk/nipple-pain/
2. The Well Project, What factors can affect HIV transmission risk during breastfeeding? https://www.thewellproject.org/hiv-information/can-i-breastfeed-while-living-hiv-overview-infant-feeding-options#What%20Factors
3. Brodribb W, Breastfeeding Management in Australia, Publishers Mothers Direct, Glen Iris, Australia
4. Smith MM and Kuhn L, Exclusive breast-feeding: does it have the potential to reduce breast-feeding transmission of HIV-1?. Nutrition Reviews 2000;58(11):333-340.
5. Coovadia HM, Rollins NC, Bland RM, Little K, Coutsoudis A, Bennish ML, Newell M-L. Mother-to-child transmission of HIV-1 infection during exclusive breastfeeding in the first 6 months of life: an intervention cohort study. Lancet 2007 March 31;369:1107-16. https://www.ncbi.nlm.nih.gov/pubmed/17398310
6. McClellan HL, Kent J C, Hepworth AR, Hartmann PE and Geddes DT, Persistent Nipple Pain in Breastfeeding Mothers Associated with Abnormal Infant Tongue Movement, Int. J. Environ. Res. Public Health 2015, 12, 10833-10845; https://www.ncbi.nlm.nih.gov/pmc/articles/PMC4586646/pdf/ijerph-12-10833.pdf
7. La Leche League Great Britain, Tongue Tie, see LLL info https://www.laleche.org.uk/tongue-tie/
8. NHS, Tongue tie https://www.nhs.uk/conditions/tongue-tie/
9. Amir L et al, Reliability of the Hazelbaker Assessment Tool for Lingual Frenulum Function, International Breastfeeding Journal, https://internationalbreastfeedingjournal.biomedcentral.com/articles/10.1186/1746-4358-1-3
10. New Zealand National Guidance for the Assessment, Diagnosis and Surgical Treatment of Tongue-tie in Breastfeeding Neonates https://www.health.govt.nz/system/files/documents/publications/national-guidance-assessment-diagnosis-surgical-treatment-tongue-tie-breastfeeding-neonates-26jan2021.pdf
11. Elad D et al, Biomechanics of milk extraction during breast-feeding, PNAS 2014, available at http://www.pnas.org/content/111/14/5230.full.pdf+html?
12. Find a Lactation Consultant through LCGB, https://lcgb.org/find-an-ibclc/

Chapter 14: Breastfeeding problems: supplementing, suspending and transitioning back

1. WHO Weight for age percentiles for boys, birth to 6 months https://cdn.who.int/media/docs/default-source/child-growth/child-growth-standards/indicators/weight-for-age/cht-wfa-boys-p-0-6.pdf?sfvrsn=2a49ab55_12
2. Weight for age percentiles for girls, birth to 6 months https://cdn.who.int/media/docs/default-source/child-growth/child-growth-standards/indicators/weight-for-age/cht-wfa-girls-p-0-6.pdf?sfvrsn=52e7206c_12
3. NHS. Your baby's weight and height, https://www.nhs.uk/conditions/baby/babys-development/height-weight-and-reviews/baby-height-and-weight/#
4. Lawrence R, (Chapter 12, Normal growth, failure to thrive, and obesity in the breastfed infant) Breastfeeding: a guide for the medical profession, 5th edition 1999, Mosby publishers.
5. Krugman, SD, and Dubowitz, H. Failure to Thrive. Am Fam Physician. 2003 Sep 1;68(5):879-884. available at http://www.aafp.org/afp/2003/0901/p879.html
6. Desmarais L and Browne S, Inadequate weight gain in breastfeeding infants; assessments and resolutions. Lactation Consultant Series Unit 8, La Leche League International.
7. The Breastfeeding Network, Contraception and breastfeeding https://www.breastfeedingnetwork.org.uk/contraception/
8. Boss M, Gardner H and Hartmann P. Normal Human Lactation: closing the gap [version 1; referees: 4 approved] F1000 Research 2018, 7(F1000 Faculty Rev):801 https://f1000research.com/articles/7-801/v1
9. La Leche League International, Mothers and Thyroidism, https://www.llli.org/breastfeeding-info/breastfeeding-and-thyroidism/#:~:text=Mothers%20with%20hypothyroidism%20are%20at,a%20negative%20effect%20on%20oxytocin.
10. Hoover K, Hoover KL, Barbalinardo LH, Platia MP. Delayed lactogenesis II secondary to gestational ovarian theca lutein cysts in two normal singleton pregnancies. J Hum Lact. 2002;18:264-268
11. Daly, SEJ, Di Rosso, A, Owens, RA, and Hartmann, PE. 1993, Degree of breast emptying explains changes in the fat content, but not fatty acid composition, of human milk, Experimental Physiology, 78:741-755.
12. The Breastfeeding Network, Domperidone and breastfeeding, https://www.breastfeedingnetwork.org.uk/wp-content/dibm/2019-09/Domperidone%20as%20a%20Galactagogue%20and%20breastfeeding.pdf .

Chapter 15: Suppression of lactation

1. BHIVA guidelines for the management of HIV in pregnancy and postpartum 2018 (2020 third interim update) https://www.bhiva.org/pregnancy-guidelines
2. BHIVA, HIV and breastfeeding your baby, Safer Triangle booklet, January 2023. https://www.bhiva.org/file/5bfd3080d2027/BF-Leaflet-1.pdf
3. European Medicines Agency, Bromocriptine-containing medicines indicated in the prevention or suppression of physiological lactation post-partum, Restrictions in use of bromocriptine for stopping breast milk production from 30 October 2014 https://www.ema.europa.eu/en/medicines/

human/referrals/bromocriptine-containing-medicines-indicated-prevention-suppression-physiological-lactation-post
4. European Multicentre Study Group for Cabergoline in Lactation Inhibition. Single dose cabergoline versus bromocriptine in inhibition of puerperal lactation. Randomised, double blind, multicentre study. BMJ 302(6789):1367-71, 1991.
5. Tulloch K et al Cabergoline: a review of its use in the inhibition of lactation for women living with HIV, JIAS 22(6) 11 June 2019 https://onlinelibrary.wiley.com/doi/full/10.1002/jia2.25322
6. Kuhn L, Kim H-Y, Walter J, Thea DM, Sinkala M, Mwiya M, Kankasa C, Decker D, Aldrovandi GM, HIV-1 Concentrations in Human Breast Milk Before and After Weaning, Sci Transl Med Vol. 5, Issue 181, p. 181ra51, Sci. Transl. Med. DOI: 10.1126/scitranslmed.3005113, Apr 2013 http://stm.sciencemag.org/content/5/181/181ra51.full.html

Chapter 16: Conclusion
1. Desmarais L & Browne S. Inadequate weight gain in breastfeeding infants; assessments and resolutions, Lactation consultant Series Unit 8, 1990 La Leche League International

INDEX

abscesses 139, 141, 148
African cultural traditions of
    breastfeeding 8–9, 11–12, 18
AIDS (Acquired Immune Deficiency
    Syndrome) 48
American Academy of Pediatrics (AAP)
    29–30, 52
antenatal preparation 40
antenatal transmission 13
antibiotics 39, 147, 148, 156
antibody testing 50
antiretroviral prophylaxis for babies 34,
    38, 49–50
antiretroviral therapy (ART) for mother
    adherence 49
    ART+EBF (antiretroviral therapy
        and exclusive breastfeeding) 20–8,
        51
    benefits of 16, 19–21
    breastfeeding after six months
        102–3
    given to babies 24
    lifelong use of 49
    preferred to ART for baby 38
    reminders to take 45
    transformational effect of 48–51
arching 67
areas of difference when breastfeeding
    with HIV 36–7
attachment (latching baby) *see* latch
    issues; latching
Australia 31
autocrine control 92

baby-led weaning 109
bacterial infection in nipples 155–6
Belgium 28
BHIVA (British HIV Association)
    breastfeeding after six months 103
    infant feeding by mothers living
        with HIV 24, 27, 28–9, 32, 50–1
    prophylactic ART for baby 38, 50
    testing recommendations 39, 49–50

when to use formula 32, 130
biological nurturing 71–2
birth, exposure to HIV during 38
birth experiences and breastfeeding
    63–4
birth-related transmission 20
biting 166
bleeding nipples 149, 152
blocked ducts 144–6
bottle-feeding
    changing from bottle to breast 81
    expressed milk 118–29
    making familiar 59–60
    nipple confusion 80
    sterilisation 122, 123
    supplementation 181
    weaning from the breast 111, 115
breast compressions 95, 142
'breast crawl' 64–5
breast problems 138–48
breast pumps 42, 125–6
breast refusal 119, 165–9
breast size and shape 117
breast tissue damage, preventing 93, 96
breastfeeding beyond six months 102–8
breastfeeding counsellors 41, 163
breastfeeding plan, making a 36, 65
breastfeeding support 40–1, 82, 161–4
breastmilk production 83–4
breastmilk-feeding (expressed milk)
    118–29
breastmilk-only diet 37
bromocriptine 188

cabbage 95–6, 143, 145, 146, 190
cabergoline 189
Canada 28
CD4 counts 24–5, 49
cereal 58
Chantry, Dr Caroline 132
Chibwesha, Carla 21
child protective services 45
C-hold 74

217

chronic condition, HIV as 48
cleft palate 87
clicking sounds 154
ClinicalInfo 30, 50
cluster feeding 46, 89, 90, 91, 99
cognitive development 105
colostrum 82, 83, 85, 119, 120, 135, 151, 171
comfort, feeding/sucking for 67, 90, 110, 111, 113, 161
confidentiality 44
contraception 112–13, 175
Coovadia, Gerry 55, 58
counselling 19, 30, 32
Coutsoudis, Anna 55
Covid-19 39
cracked nipples 154–5
cradle hold 68
cross-cradle hold 69–70
crying 67, 153, 167, 177
cultural norms 8–9, 11–12, 18
cup feeding 95, 118, 127, 181

definitions
  antenatal transmission 13
  breastfeeding 14–15
  exclusive breastfeeding 20, 22–3, 52
  exclusive breastfeeding for the first six months of life 55
  important 13–15
  vertical transmission (VT) 13
delayed first breastfeed 65
delayed lactation 96–7
demand-led feeding 88, 89, 90–1, 94, 96, 98–9, 175, 177
depression 189, 190
diarrhoea 130
disclosure of HIV status 44
domperidone 183, 185
donor milk 30, 134
dummies 42, 111, 161, 177
duration of feeds 88, 89–90, 175

Elad, David 157–8
electrolytes 54

emergency situations 122, 133–4
emotional benefits of breastfeeding 106, 111, 113
engorgement 42, 78–9, 91–6, 115, 120, 138–47, 151–2, 189
Enhanced Register 35
epithelial barrier 55
exclusive breastfeeding for the first six months of life 20, 52–60
expressing milk 82, 95, 115–16, 118–29, 138, 143, 190

'failure to thrive' (FTT)/'faltering growth' 104, 174–5, 180
feedback inhibitor of lactation (FIL) 98, 140, 188
feeding intervals 9, 47, 89, 90–1, 98 *see also* feeding on demand
feeding on demand 88, 89, 90–1, 94, 96, 98–9, 175, 177
fertility, returning 110, 112–13
finger-feeding 129, 181
first hour after birth 64–5
flash-heating breastmilk 119, 130–6
flipple 78
fluid intake (mother's) 126, 182, 189
flutter-sucking 178
food sensitivities 100, 168
football hold/rugby hold 70–1
formula feeding
  BHIVA recommendations on using 32, 130
  gut integrity 134
  mixed feeding as risk factor for HIV transmission 93
  norm in UK 53
  offered free in 1990s 19
  stigmatised 18
  supplementation 169, 178–87
  switching to 115
  usually recommended 32, 48
  usually recommended in First World settings 18, 29
  as Western cultural norm 9
'fourth trimester' 63

INDEX

freezing milk 122, 126, 136, 192
frenotomies 37, 82, 133, 157–8, 176
frequency of feeds 90–1, 175 *see also* feeding on demand

galactagogues 183, 185
gastroenteritis 53, 130
Germany 27
global guidance *see also* WHO recommendations
   breastfeeding after six months 103
   infant feeding 16, 28, 52
   reversals in 9, 19, 55
Global Health Media 78
grief 113, 189, 190
growth factors 55, 103
gut integrity 15, 20, 21, 55–6, 102, 133, 134, 194

HAART (Highly Active Antiretroviral Therapy) 21
hand-expressing 95, 119–20, 123–4, 138
'happy to starve' babies 91
health visitors 36, 100, 174
healthcare professionals 34–5, 36, 42–3, 53 *see also* paediatricians
high muscle tone 178
HIV clinicians 33–4
HIV Kit 13
HIV levels in milk 93, 120, 146
HIV status, disclosure of 44
Holder pasteurisation 131–2
horizontal transmission 25
hormonal birth control 175
hormones in lactogenesis 84–5 *see also* oxytocin; prolactin
hospital discharge 41
hospital-grade double electric breast pumps 42, 125–6
Human Milk Banking Association of North America 132

IABLE 78
IBCLCs 41, 82, 161, 163, 170

Iliff, Dr Peter 20
immunological components of being close to mother 88
immunological components of breastmilk 50, 83, 106, 122, 132
inadequate glandular breast tissue 176
indicators of successful breastfeeding 99–101 *see also* urine / stool output; weight gain
Infant Feeding Survey (2010) 53
inflammation 20, 57, 102, 141, 143, 146
informed choice 33
initiation of breastmilk production 84–6
international guidelines 9, 16, 19, 28 *see also* WHO recommendations
intervals between feeds 9, 47, 89, 90–1, 98
intestinal epithelial barrier 55
iron 175
ISOSS (Integrated Screening Outcomes Surveillance Service) 27, 35, 107

'jarring' 150–1
jaundice 91, 176–7
Jeffery, Bridget 132

koala hold 71
Kuhn, Louise 55–6
kwashiorkor 111

La Leche League 11, 12, 41, 106
lactation consultants 34, 36, 41, 82, 161, 163, 170
Lactation Consultants of Great Britain 41
lactogenesis 84–6, 97
laid-back breastfeeding 71–2
latch issues 78–9, 81–2, 149, 151, 152
latching 67, 73–80, 151–3, 162
learning to breastfeed 62–3
legal counsel 44–5
length of feeds 88, 89–90, 175
let-down reflex 86
lip ties 157–8

219

lipstick-shaped nipples 154
low weight gain 100, 169, 173–87

making the choice to breastfeed 33
malnutrition 111
massaging the breasts 95, 123, 143, 145, 190
mastitis 39, 57, 91–2, 110, 119, 133, 139, 141, 145–7, 192
medications (other than ART)
   affecting baby's latch 78–9
   antibiotics 147, 148, 156
   during birth 64
   counting as 'mixed feeding' 37
   galactagogues 185
   hormonal birth control 100, 175
   suppression of lactation 188–9
meta-analyses 22
milk banks 131–2
milk failing to come in 96–7
milk fat 88
'milk fever' 189
milk stasis 57, 110, 141
milk transfer to baby 86–9
milk-ejection reflex 86, 141
milk-producing cells 42, 91, 93–4, 97, 141, 191
Minchin, Maureen 134
mixed feeding
   after six months 102–8
   compromised gut integrity 54–6
   effect on quality of breastmilk 57
   effect on risk of HIV transmission 54–5
   gut integrity 55–6
Morrison, P. 140
mothering the mother 45–6, 101
mothering tools 63, 67, 106
mother-led weaning 109, 115
mother-to-child transmission (MTCT) 13, 26, 48, 51
multidisciplinary teams 32, 34–5, 106–7, 156, 170
muscle tone 88, 178

naloxone 78–9
nappies, as indicators of successful feeding 99, 113, 171, 176–7, 184
National Perinatal HIV Hotline 35
negative pressure 151
nevirapine 38
New Zealand 31, 51
Newman, Dr Jack 87
night-time feeding 101
nipple abrasions 154
nipple confusion 80, 128, 186
nipple pointing upwards technique 76
nipple problems 149–64
nipple sandwich 77–8
nipple shields 82, 159–60
'not enough milk' 93, 96–7, 169, 171
nursing pillows 68
nursing strikes 119, 165–9
nutritional content of breastmilk 53–4, 105, 111, 121, 122, 182

obstetricians 36
oedema 143
oestrogen 84
oral suctioning 36
overfeeding 88
over-fullness 57, 86, 91–6, 120, 138–47, 151–2
overproduction of milk 121, 139, 140
oxytocin 86, 87, 125, 141

paced bottle-feeding 128
pacifiers 42, 111, 161, 177
paediatricians
   lack of understanding of breastfeeding 9
   low weight gain 170, 174, 185
   sharing your breastfeeding plan with 36
parsley 144
pasteurising breastmilk 115, 119, 122, 130–6, 144, 181
pethidine 64, 78–9
placenta 84, 85, 97, 175
plan, making a 36, 59

polycystic ovarian syndrome 176
porridge 53, 58
positional sore stripe 154
positioning for breastfeeding 65–73, 149–51
post-exposure prophylaxis (PEP) 49–50
postpartum haemorrhage 175
postpartum transmission (PP transmission) 14
pre-chewed food 108
pregnancy-associated transmission 14
premature exposure to foreign substances 20
prenatal transmission *see* antenatal transmission
pre-term babies 11–12, 139
professional breastfeeding support 163
progesterone 84, 85, 97
prolactin 85, 94, 97, 101, 141, 189, 190
PROMISE study 23, 24
Public Health England 27
pumping milk 42, 119–20, 125–6, 138, 143

reflexes 66–7, 86, 104
re-latching 152–3
research methodologies 21–8
resting nipples 160–1
retained placenta 97, 175
risk of antenatal transmission 13
risk of birth-related transmission 20
risk of breastfeeding-associated transmission
    ART+EBF (antiretroviral therapy and exclusive breastfeeding) reduces risk to virtually zero 51
    balancing with risk of other diseases 103
    breast pathology 145
    breastfeeding after six months 14, 102–3
    and child's gut maturity 103
    duration of ART 21
    engorgement 91–6, 141–2, 145, 191–2

    exclusive breastfeeding for the first six months of life 14
    formula supplementation 180
    frenotomies 158
    global guidance 16–17
    'ideal scenario' conditions for minimal risk 106–7
    importance of ART in reducing 21, 48–9, 51
    increased by mixed feeding 55, 180
    mastitis 146
    mixed breastfeeding after six months 14
    pasteurisation/flash-heating of breastmilk 130–6
    premature exposure to foreign substances 14
    reducing to virtually nil 18, 51
    remains lower even after exclusive breastfeeding period ends 54–5
    research background 18–19
    sore nipples 149, 161
risk of transmission with pre-chewed food 108
risks of not breastfeeding 18, 33
Royal College of Paediatricians 174
rugby hold/football hold 70–1

sage 144
saggy breasts 117
scissors hold 77
separation of mother and baby after birth 37, 57
shared decision-making 30, 31, 32–3
sick babies 130, 139
side-lying breastfeeding positions 72–3
skin-to-skin after birth 36, 64–5
sleep 67, 101, 111–12
slow weaning 191
Smith, Melanie 55–6
solicitors 45
solid food, starting
    developmental readiness for 104
    early introduction raises risk of transmission 55

nutritional content 110–11
as preparation for weaning from breast 110
risks of pre-chewed food 108
waiting until 6 months 38, 54
sore nipples 118–19, 139, 149–64, 176
South Africa 55, 132
spoon feeding 95, 118, 127, 181
sterilisation 121, 123, 126
stimulating baby to open mouth 73–4
stools, as indicators of successful feeding 99, 113, 184
stopping breastfeeding at six months 102–3
stopping breastfeeding, planning in advance 42 *see also* weaning from the breast
storage capacity of breasts 83–4, 90, 92, 97, 99
storing expressed breastmilk 121–2, 144
storing pasteurised breastmilk 135–6
'stunting' 178
sub-clinical mastitis 145–7
suck training 80
sucking and swallowing, effective 87–9, 95
sucking needs 59, 111, 128, 161
sulpride 185
supplemental nursing systems 129, 181
supplementation 178–87
support
　breastfeeding support 40–1, 82, 161–4
　for mothers dealing with low weight gain 185
　for new mothers 45–6, 101
supporting the breast during feeding 74–9, 153, 162–3
suppression of lactation 188–93
Swiss Statement 25, 26
Switzerland 27
syringe feeding 129

Tanzania 26, 102, 132
tea 125
tea-cup hold 78–9
testing
　antibody testing 39
　of baby 34, 37, 38–9, 49–50
　bacterial infection in nipples 156
　during cases of mastitis 39
　mastitis 147
　viral load 34, 37, 38
　viral testing of breastmilk 39
theca-luteinising cysts 176
theophylline 125
thrush 133, 156–7
thyroid functioning 175–6
ties (e.g. tongue, lip) 37, 157–8
tight junctions 57, 91, 93, 141, 190
tongue ties 37, 43, 81–2, 157–8, 176
transitioning back to breastfeeding 45, 81, 128, 134, 182, 186

UK National Breastfeeding Helpline 41
UK national HIV and infant feeding recommendations 28–9 *see also* BHIVA (British HIV Association)
UK NOURISH 107
UNAIDS 19
undetectable=untransmittable (u=u) for horizontal transmission 24–5
undetectable=untransmittable (u=u) for vertical transmission 26
unexplained breast pain 148
unhappy babies 100
UNICEF guidance 17, 19
unlatching 161
urine/stool output 99, 113, 171, 176–7, 184
US Panel on Treatment of HIV in Pregnancy and Prevention of Perinatal Transmission 30, 32
USA 28, 29–30, 35, 50, 51

Vernazza, Pietro 26
vertical transmission (VT) 13, 26

INDEX

viral load 21, 24, 25, 27, 34, 49, 102–3
visitors, dealing with 47
vomiting 130

water 53, 54, 55, 58
water content of breastmilk 54, 89
weaning from the breast 109–17
   abrupt 103, 111, 115–16
   practical strategies 113–14
   slow weaning 116
   suppression of lactation 188–93
weaning grief 113, 189, 190
weight charts 53, 99–100
weight checks (baby) 38, 40
weight gain 40, 99–100, 126, 169, 172–87 *see also* low weight gain
WHO Code 12
WHO Interagency Task Team 103

WHO recommendations
   antiretroviral prophylaxis for babies 38
   breastfeeding after six months 103, 105
   breastfeeding recommendations 52, 54
   infant feeding by mothers living with HIV 16, 17, 19, 50–1, 109
   prophylactic ART for baby 50
   solid food recommendation 108
   weight charts 53, 99–100, 172
World Alliance for Breastfeeding Action (WABA) 13

Zambia 21, 58, 102
Zimbabwe 11–12, 20, 55, 132
ZVITAMBO project 20, 55, 132–3

Also by Pamela Morrison

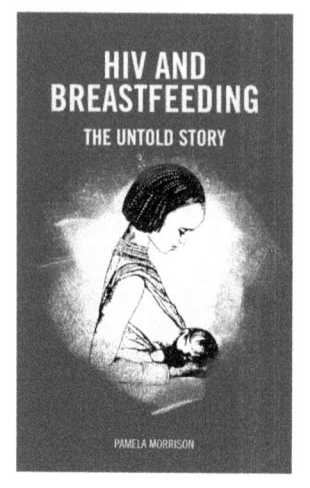

In the early 1980s it was discovered that HIV, the virus that causes AIDS, could be passed through a mother's milk to her baby. Almost overnight in the industrialised countries, and later in the African countries most ravaged by HIV, breastfeeding became an endangered practice. But in the rush to reduce transmission of HIV, everything we already knew about breastfeeding's life-saving effects was overlooked, with devastating consequences for mothers and babies.

In *HIV and Breastfeeding: the untold story*, former IBCLC Pamela Morrison, an acknowledged authority on HIV and breastfeeding, reveals how women in the world's most poverty-stricken areas were persuaded to abandon breastfeeding as part of a short-sighted and deadly policy that led to a humanitarian disaster. The dilemma that breastfeeding, an act of nurturing which confers food, comfort and love, could be at once life-saving yet lethal, has been called 'the ultimate paradox'. This critical account reveals how vital breastfeeding is, even in the most difficult of circumstances, and examines the lessons that can be learned from the mistakes of the past – which is particularly relevant as we deal with the consequences for mothers and babies of another global pandemic, Covid-19.

With detailed information for HIV-positive mothers and their caregivers, and success stories from mothers themselves, this book is essential reading for anyone involved in protecting and supporting breastfeeding, or with a need for evidence-based information about breastfeeding and HIV.

HIV and Breastfeeding: the untold story
2022 | paperback | ISBN: 9781780667508

Milton Keynes UK
Ingram Content Group UK Ltd.
UKHW020731260424
441811UK00014B/731